# NURSING AUXILIARIES IN HEALTH CARE

# NURSING AUXILIARIES IN HEALTH CARE

Edited by MELISSA HARDIE and LISBETH HOCKEY

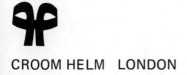

CROOM HELM   LONDON

Croom Helm Ltd, 2-10 St John's Road, London SW11

British Library Cataloguing in Publication Data

Nursing auxiliaries in health care.
　　1. Nurses' aides
　　I. Hardie, Melissa　II. Hockey, Lisbeth
　　610.73'0698　　　R T84

　　ISBN 0-85664-529-X

Printed and bound in Great Britain by
Billing & Sons Limited, Guildford, London and Worcester

# CONTENTS

To the memory of
PROFESSOR SIR HUGH ROBSON 1917-77
Vice Chancellor of the University of Edinburgh
and friend to us

# FOREWORD

It is becoming increasingly evident that throughout Europe and North America the health service boom of the post-war era is over. Irrespective of whether its health service is nationalised or pluralistic, socialised or commercialised, no country can any longer afford to allow expenditure on health services to continue increasing at an annual rate considerably greater than the annual growth in gross national product.

Staff costs account for around two-thirds of the total health service budget in most countries. It is therefore not surprising that manpower planning and research are of increasing interest and importance to all health service authorities, along with questions of cost containment, monitoring of services and quality control. Likewise, with nursing staff forming the largest component part of total health manpower, it is also not surprising that nursing research is becoming of particular significance to those responsible for the planning and management of health services.

Against this background, it is very understandable that the current research project of the Nursing Research Unit of the University of Edinburgh on nursing auxiliaries should be of immediate practical interest to the planners and managers who make up the bulk of the membership of the International Hospital Federation. The IHF was therefore very glad to have the opportunity of collaborating with the Nursing Research Unit (itself a corporate member of the IHF) in organising an international workshop in Edinburgh to discuss the progress of the Unit's research project with representatives from Britain and thirteen other countries in Europe and North America. It is the papers presented and discussed at this workshop that form the basis of this book.

Reflecting upon these papers and upon the discussion at the seminar, one is struck by the variety of staffing patterns and training programmes that have been developed by different countries to prepare staff to meet the needs of patients for bedside and domestic care. These needs do not vary much in kind from one country to another, but the methods of meeting these needs show surprising differences. Most countries provide a training of around three years for state registration as a nurse; but for assistant nurses and nursing

9

auxiliaries or helpers, it seems that training can last anything from two weeks to two years. Confusion is compounded by semantic and philosophical differences within and between countries over the relative roles and responsibilities of nurses and auxiliaries. This brings to mind Florence Nightingale's comment nearly a hundred years ago in 1882, when she said that 'A good nurse of 20 years ago had not to do the twentieth part of what she is required by her physician or surgeon to do now.'

We are faced with similar problems today, and the importance of matching people to jobs was neatly summarised in a report from the United States of America in 1967, which drew attention to 'the dangerous practice of assigning people to tasks for which they are undertrained and the wasteful practice of assigning people to tasks for which they are overtrained.' It is hoped that the papers presented in this book will help to clarify some of the important issues involved in the recruitment, training, deployment of nurses and auxiliaries and thus help to make a contribution to knowledge and understanding of problems that are of widespread concern to all those involved in the provision of health services.

Miles Hardie
Director-General
International Hospital Federation

# PREFACE

The proportion of auxiliaries in nursing (less than fully qualified
nursing personnel) has until very recently been increasing steadily
within the hospital and community health services in Britain. It may be
levelling out currently and perhaps even decreasing due to the
competitive labour market in which the professionally qualified, as in
many other fields, are vying for employment. However, little critical
attention has been paid to the arrangements for employing, deploying
and preparing these workers in developed countries for their demanding
and important contribution to health care, while the 'specialisation
phenomenon' continues to expand for the professionals. Where are the
cutting edges in the division of labour in health care?

Both specialty and general care workers are required in most health
services. How is the place for the auxiliary defined and with what
measures of flexibility? Training resources must be universally available
but not wasted. How can the disciplines of management, economics,
nursing, medicine and the social sciences help achieve appropriate staff
balances for various health care environments? The special purpose
of this workshop was to bring together people from within these
disciplines to attempt to compare systems and changes internationally
in the use of auxiliary personnel, and to draw out lessons relevant to
our home countries.

The form of the workshop was made up of seven half-day sessions
over four working days in addition to an evening open discussion.
Eight set conference papers were delivered interspersed with nine
shorter case papers from various countries. Working groups met each
day to discuss four topics related to auxiliary employment: training;
team integration; supervision; and organisational models for the future.
Summaries of these working group sessions appear in the text together
with the general summation made on the final day by Professor
A. Altschul, of the University of Edinburgh. The sessions were held at
the university, and were organised by the Nursing Research Unit there
in collaboration with the International Hospital Federation.

In 1956, a Nursing Studies Unit was formed at the University of
Edinburgh, which was recognised as a university department in 1965.
The first professorial chair in nursing in Britain was established in 1972.
In the progress of the Nursing Studies Department's work, the

need for a research unit developed to: (a) research into nursing problems; (b) promote educational activities related to research; and (c) collect and disseminate information. From the appointment of its first director, Miss Lisbeth Hockey, in 1971, the Nursing Research Unit has undertaken this remit.

The International Hospital Federation (IHF) is an independent, non-political body whose aims are to promote improvements in the planning and management of hospitals and health services. Under its current name it was re-incorporated under Swiss law in 1947, after a cessation of activities during the war years. Originally established in 1928, the Federation has a long history of international and regional congresses and conferences, study tours in various countries, research projects and health administration educational activities. It maintains an information service for members and publishes a quarterly journal, *World Hospitals*. Some seventy countries have members in the IHF.

The research project which first stimulated interest in sponsoring a meeting about this topic was 'The Nursing Auxiliary in the National Health Service'. It was funded jointly by the Scottish Home and Health Department and the Department of Health and Social Security. Interim findings of this study are reported in one of the following set papers, and this descriptive study was concluded in January 1978. Further work is currently funded until mid-1980, with particular reference to the nursing auxiliary in the mental health and community health services.

# ACKNOWLEDGEMENTS

The organisers would like to thank Miss Margaret Auld, Chief Nursing Officer of the Scottish Home and Health Department, Dr E.V. Kuenssberg, President of the Royal College of General Practitioners, and Professor Sir Hugh Robson, Principal and Vice-Chancellor of the University of Edinburgh, for their warm addresses of welcome to the participants. Also, to Dr Monnica Stewart and Mr Arthur Thwaites for their spirited leadership of the evening discussion. Mrs Maureen Ross, secretary to the Nursing Auxiliary Research Project, was largely responsible for the administration of the meeting. The Johnson & Johnson Company and the Bank of Scotland contributed financially to the workshop.

PART ONE:
THE ROLE OF THE NURSING AUXILIARY

# 1  AUXILIARIES AND THE HEALTH CARE TEAM: THE INTERNATIONAL SCENE

Katherine Elliott

During this last year I have sensed everywhere a growing concern about gaps in health care and a realisation that highly trained health professionals (the doctors and the nurses) cannot meet the health needs of any country on their own. They must rely upon appropriate assistance from less highly trained people, however difficult they find it to share responsibility. The whole greater profession of medicine — doctors, nurses, midwives, dentists, veterinarians, sanitary engineers, pharmacists, health inspectors, radiographers, laboratory technicians, physiotherapists, and so on — we all of us face the same territorial dilemmas. If we look together at both the opportunities and the difficulties, this may help us all. Ours is a common goal: a healthier world. Hand in hand we are likely to arrive there sooner than we will if we have to contend with unnecessary barriers among ourselves.

The obvious growing world interest in the potential contribution of auxiliaries pleases me greatly, for I have been thinking for quite a long time about the problem of how to provide health care for those who have so little or nothing at all — the poorest people in the poorest countries. In 1975 Mr McNamara talked to the World Bank's Board of Governors about the 700 million rural poor and the 200 million urban poor who, as he put it, live 'in a degree of deprivation. . .so extreme as to be an insult to human dignity'. Two years have passed since he gave those figures. One thing about which we can be sure is that they have not diminished. The poor in 1977 are greater in number and they have even less. A quarter of the world's population, one out of every four human beings alive on this planet, remains trapped within a vicious circle of poverty, ignorance, disease, malnutrition and wretched surroundings and receives little or no advantage from all the advances that have been made in scientific and biomedical knowledge and skills. Population pressures continue to increase. Energy costs soar even higher. Food prices rise and current agricultural practices need a lot of rethinking. Industrial growth, if thought of in terms of high technology and on a massive scale, benefits whom? Are not all of us beginning to ask this question, and in the developing countries the squalor of the peri-urban slums supplies a discouraging clue to the probable answer: few benefit as things are now.

So the problem remains gigantic and, although we may be solving bits of it as our knowledge increases, new and unpredictable difficulties constantly arise. So-called civilisation may bring some benefits to health: its different stresses also bring new health problems. And expectations for health and well-being are everywhere on the increase as communications extend and expand and more people have access to at least some kind of formal education. In an era when television viewers sitting comfortably at home in London, Paris, Washington, Ottawa, Tokyo, Stockholm, Sydney, Brussels, Bonn and Edinburgh can now watch people dying from hunger and disease in less fortunate parts of the world, such preventable deaths are no longer accepted as an inevitable pa of human existence. And we should not forget that the communication media are not one-way mirrors. Transistor radios are as ubiquitous as chewing-gum, cornflakes and Coca Cola. Television screens in shop windows and in bars and eating places in every town and city fascinate those who have so little else that is bright in their lives. The poor everywhere have a more realistic appreciation of their own degree of deprivation and are starting to demand the chance of a better life for themselves.

What is to be done about this widening gap? It cannot be ignored either at country level or at world level. There are two obvious barriers to the improvement of world health. These are: lack of health professionals and lack of money to spend on health care. No one doubts that more doctors and nurses are needed in very many countries, but their education is expensive. They must be used, like all other scarce and costly resources, in the right places and in the right way to provide the maximum satisfaction for everyone, including the health professionals themselves.

The Director-General of the World Health Organisation, Dr Halfdan Mahler, has suggested that medical education as at present orientated tends to turn out doctors who are 'socially irrelevant'. He may be right, and a lot of thought is being devoted to finding ways of changing conventional medical training. We are conscious that medical schools in developing countries which have taken famous schools in the Western world as models produce what Professor Fendall calls 'elegantly trained physicians' who are unhappy when they are asked to work in the 'inelegant situations' where medical care is most needed. I suspect that the nursing profession is suffering the same crisis of reappraisal. What would Florence Nightingale have recommended, I wonder, if she were alive today? Her breadth of vision was immense, seeing as she did how important for health were such matters as clean water, unpolluted air, a decent diet, adequate shelter, satisfying leisure pursuits and a mind at ease. She said: 'Health is not only to be well, but to be able to use well every power we have to use.' Her description reminds us of Ivan Illich, who describes health as the state of being able to cope successfully with life, and his accusation that the medical establishment has become a major threat to health cannot be lightly dismissed.

Sir Theodore Fox, formerly Editor of the *Lancet,* asked in 1956: 'Have we, I wonder, sufficiently adjusted ourselves to the change that is coming over medicine?' He commented: 'For the normal tendency of a service is to turn all its members into employees working by the rule – to destroy rather than foster their feeling that they are members of free professions.' Twenty-one years ago this wise man, who coined the term 'the greater medical profession' to embrace all of us who take care of people's health, saw the need for a change of heart. In the interim, the need he foresaw has become still more urgent for social and political, as well as medical, reasons – for some of the harm he feared has surely come to pass. The health professionals are much less sure of their roles and how they should relate to each other. The health professions, by their very nature, tend anyway to be resistant to change – and their conservatism varies greatly from country to country.

Let me turn for a moment to the implications of one interesting experiment among the many taking place in various parts of the world in which a good deal of health care is being provided by people with minimal training. David Werner is a biologist who found himself setting up a village health project in the remote mountains of Mexico where no health professionals were available and where there is still no resident doctor. This has worked so well that the village people can now manage without even David himself, and they feel capable of seeding off similar projects in adjoining needy areas. David Werner spoke at the International Hospital Federation Congress in Japan earlier this year and his message was that the health professional, if world health needs are to be met, must move into the position of being 'on tap' instead of being 'on top'. This means that the pyramid of medical responsibility topples sideways to expose the maximum interface to the surrounding community so that people can understand the part played in their lives by health-related matters and can make their own personal contributions in an enlightened and responsible fashion. Because health professionals move from the centre of the

stage into the wings, with corresponding changes in the roles they play
in the actual delivery of health care services, this does not release
them from the burden of being finally accountable, of the need to be
always 'on tap' through channels which they must help to set up.
Wise parents do not try to stop their children from going out in the
rain, but they do make sure they know what an umbrella is for — and
they keep a supply of umbrellas handy for the children to use: and a
back-up service of dry towels and hot baths! I will come back again to
this question of accountability, but first I want to venture a little
further into the auxiliary arena.

When I say that the world picture of the health of the people is still
sombre but that, despite the fact that it is getting worse in many places,
there are nevertheless some encouraging signs, I am talking about the
growing world interest in the potential of auxiliary health care
personnel and about the intriguing innovative projects which are
gradually becoming better known, such as David Werner's in Mexico.
The idea of health care auxiliaries is far from a new one. There have
always been persons in the community with an interest in caring for the
sick and with some particular skill to offer to whom the people in need
turned in the days when doctors were rare and trained nurses
non-existent. There have been — and still are — traditional healers and
birth attendants, shamans, bone-setters, wise women and herbalists.

And we should not forget how, in our own society, people ask
for advice from anyone who works on the drug counter in a chemist's
shop, not just the pharmacist or the dispenser, and from anyone who
works in a hospital or in a general practitioner's surgery, not just the
doctor or the nurse. They ask older colleagues, schoolteachers and
clergymen. They even write to magazines and ring up radio chat
programmes. People consult a whole variety of sources about what to
do when they are bothered about their health. They do not
necessarily feel that only a doctor or a nurse can provide acceptable
advice. If the problem continues or is obviously something serious,
they seek out a health professional but, for simple ailments,
people do recognise that others who may have picked up a little
useful knowledge and perhaps had a lot of experience may be able to
help them quite satisfactorily without any form of special training in
health care.

In Austria in the eighteenth century, the physician Johann Peter
Frank thought it a good idea to equip the parish priests with medical
supplies. Peter the Great sent the army medical orderlies off to become
the first feldschers in the country districts of Russia. There is a long and

honourable tradition among medical missionaries that they should train medical assistants. Colonial medical services formalised the concept with such institutions as the Fiji Medical School, which trained a local practitioner. India had its Licensed Medical Practitioners, licensed to work in India only. Sudan and Nigeria have a long history of the medical assistant who was part of a team which spread out to the village aid post orderly.

But no one suggested that the auxiliary concept could formally apply in a Western country. It was unlawful for anyone with less than the full professional training to meddle with health care: we remained convinced that our conventional patterns of medical care, hospital-based and provided only through professionals with long and expensive training, was the best way to do it. And if the health care the poor in our own country received happened to be rather makeshift at times, how sad, but we were sure it would all be perfect eventually when we could afford more doctors, more nurses and more hospitals.

That day is very far off for most countries, and meanwhile people have been experimenting with a wide variety of alternatives, compelled by necessity and urged on by the realisation that Fendall's elegantly trained professionals, whom I mentioned earlier, are not always at their best in inelegant situations for which their training has failed to equip them. The auxiliary, who may work either full- or part-time, acts as a partial alternative to the full health professional. The responsibilities of auxiliaries are defined by the tasks they perform rather than by traditional professional roles. Their training is primarily oriented to the work they will undertake, rather than being based upon a wide background of theoretical knowledge as in conventional medical, nursing and paramedical education. Their authority is derived from the public or private health care organisation within which the auxiliary works, rather than from the traditional professional licensing bodies. This suggested description of an auxiliary stresses the task-oriented team focus to the work of auxiliaries in health care and the need to relate levels of competence — or what Dr Ed Pellegrino has called 'the allowable amount of discretionary space' — to the particular situations being met.

Having tried to describe auxiliaries, I want to go further out into the arena and ask why we have so much trouble with this noun. The World Health Organisation's definition of an auxiliary is 'a technical worker in a certain field with less than the full professional qualification'. This in no way helps to offset the demeaning connotation which springs, I suspect, from the Latin word 'auxiliar' which had a military and frequently pejorative significance — Caesar and his generals regarded auxiliaries as unreliable, lacking as they did the proper Roman training and discipline. But we ought to remember that local troops with very little training, but who know the countryside well, may cope better in some tricky situations. The roots of the word go further back to the Greek root 'auxein', which means to increase. Therefore to me the auxiliary is not just a helpful bystander to the professional — an assistant or an ancillary — but someone with a proper degree of autonomy who can increase and enlarge the outreach of the professional and carry part of the load independently.

Words are important, and they change in meaning. T.S. Eliot wrote: 'Words strain, crack and sometimes break under the burden, under the tension, slip, slide, perish, decay with imprecision, will not stay in place, will not stay still.' It could be useful to look again at some of the words we bandy about so readily and think again about their meaning. I believe we tend to hide real issues behind semantic arguments, like squids which conceal themselves in clouds of sepia ink. This applies very much to this awkward noun 'auxiliary', which I have just tried to rehabilitate. We talk about health care, not medical care and nursing care. We talk about the caring professions. We talk very little about taking care of people and how everyone can share in taking care of others. Muriel Skeet reminded me one day how very good undertakers are at taking care, not only of the dead, but also of the living who are bereaved.

Another dubious word is 'role'. We, the so-called health professionals, talk about our roles, as if we are actors and can become different people off-stage. Can we really do this? We may need to carry out David Werner's suggestion and step away from the centre of the stage into the wings, but the play never stops and we have no understudies.

Just to add to the semantic jungle, I suggest a new noun: 'the healthmasters'. Health has become a big industry; and I was thinking recently about the Industrial Revolution and that word that had so much significance then: 'the ironmasters' — the men with the knowledge, the power, the resources and the enterprise who were the founders of modern industrial society. I see a rapidly growing equivalent: the 'healthmasters', who could, if they wished, inspire the development of a healthier world society. The healthmasters are not just the health professionals in the original meaning — the doctors, the nurses, the paramedicals — like, for example, pharmacists, radiographers, therapists of all kinds and so on but, equally important, the administrators and managers, and the whole new breed of health

planners, health economists, architects and designers — people often
without real contact with any direct form of care-giving, but whose
decisions profoundly affect the shape of health services. I don't
think the old ironmasters knew what the total effect of their
industries would be on the lives of the communities involved. I think
we need to be careful that the new healthmasters know exactly
what they are doing to people.

I find it encouraging that people are beginning to take another
long hard look at health care in the West and to wonder whether we
are, after all, getting value for our money. It is not just a question
of whether we can any longer afford the escalating costs of the National
Health Service: it is also a question of whether the Service is meeting
all the needs of all of the people. We speak about the health team.
Health teams begin with the people themselves, who are after all the
greatest resource we have. The healthmasters are accountable for the
success of health teams because it is their knowledge and expertise
which must be appropriately shared down through their auxiliary
counterparts in order to reach every family. By sharing responsibility
we can make the work that only we can do more effective. As Dr
Maurice King wrote in 1975: 'In our age the greatest challenge
before world medicine is to see that the most useful parts of the
knowledge *we already have* are brought to all those who need it'.
But we cannot avoid the final accountability because we must, being
who we are, always decide what the safe levels of competence are
and be ready to come to the rescue when needed. Thinking
about accountability, I remember very well how I recognised, as a
medical student on the wards, what must be rendered unto Caesar
and what unto God. One was the consultant and one was the ward
sister: I leave you to imagine which I thought of as which.

There is unfortunately no fear that the world will soon have no
further use for doctors, nurses and other health care experts, that
the greater medical profession will pass into limbo. But the trend on
the international scene towards the development of a wide variety of
health workers, some of whom have received only a minimal training
and who remain very much part of the community, cannot be
disregarded. We have exported our conventional system of health
care and this has left two-thirds of the world almost untouched. It
could be that we can now perhaps learn something for our own
benefit from the Third World and its experiments with unconventional
ways of taking care of its health problems.

## Bibliography

Adamson, T. Elaine. 'Critical Issues in the Use of Physician Associates and Assistants'. AJPH Vol.61, No.9, 1971, pp.1765-79.

Lord Ashby of Brandon. 'Protection of the Environment: The Human Dimension'. (Jephcott Lecture) *Proc. R. Soc. Medicine,* London, Vol.69, 1976, pp.721-30.

Behrhorst, C. The Chimaltenango Development Project. *Contact* No.19, Christian Medical Commission of World Council of Churches, Geneva, 1974.

Bicknell, William J., Chapman Walsh, Diana and Tanner, Marsha M. 'Substantial or Decorative? Physicians' Assistants and Nurse Practitioners in the United States'. *The Lancet,* No.7891, 1974, pp.1241-44.

Chamberlain, R.W. and Radebaugh, J.F. 'Delivery of Primary Health Care – Union Style (A critical review of the Robert F. Kennedy Plan for the United Farm Workers of America). *New England J. of Medicine,* Vol.294, No.12, pp.641-5.

Elliott, Katherine. 'Using Medical Auxiliaries: Some Ideas and Examples' in *Health Manpower and the Medical Auxiliary.* Intermediate Technology Publications, London, 1971, pp.29-46. Reprinted as *Contact,* No.11, Christian Medical Commission of World Council of Churches, Geneva, 1972. (Also available in French and Spanish.)

—— 'Meeting World Health Needs: The Doctor and the Medical Auxiliary' in *World Hospitals,* 1973. Reprinted in *World Medical Journal,* Vol.23, No.3, May/June 1976.

—— *The Training of Auxiliaries in Health Care: An Annotated Bibliography.* Intermediate Technology Publications, London, 1975, p.110.

—— 'The Year of the Health Auxiliary?' in *British Health Care Planning & Technology.* Year Book of the British Hospitals Export Council, London, 1975.

—— 'Towards Fairer Play in the World Health Game'. International Health Soc. Bulletin. Oxon Hill, Maryland, April 1976.

—— 'The Rest of the Health Team'. Proc. of International Conference on *Priorities for the Use of Resources in Medicine.* Fogarty International Center, Bethesda, Maryland, November 1976.

—— 'The Health Auxiliary: An Example of Appropriate Health Technology' in *Internationale Entwicklung (International Development).* Austrian Foundation for Development Research, Vienna, 1977.

—— 'Do Doctors Sometimes Suffer from High Altitude Problems?' in *Health Auxiliaries and the Health Team.* Proc. XXth International Hospital Federation Congress in Tokyo, May 1977. Croom Helm, London (forthcoming).

—— 'Auxiliaries and Health Teams: The International Scene' in *Auxiliaries in Health Care: Case Studies in Nursing.* Proc. International Workshop on Nursing Auxiliaries organised by the International Hospital Federation in Edinburgh, September 1977. Croom Helm, London (forthcoming).

—— (ed.) *The Family and its Future.* (Ciba Found. Symp.), Churchill Livingstone, Edinburgh, 1970, p.230.

Elliott, Katherine and FitzSimons, D.W. (eds.) *Breast-feeding and the Mother.* (Ciba Found. Symp. 45), Elsevier/Excerpta Medica/North Holland, Amsterdam and New York, 1976, p.288.

Elliott, Katherine and Knight, Julie (eds.) *Acute Diarrhoea in Childhood.* (Ciba Found. Symp. 42), Elsevier/Excerpta Medica/North Holland, Amsterdam and New York, 1976, p.384.

Elliott, Katherine and Whelan, Julie (eds.) *Health and Disease in Tribal Societies.* (Ciba Found. Symp.49), Elsevier/Excerpta Medica/North Holland, Amsterdam and New York, 1977, p.344.
—— *Health and Industrial Growth.* (Ciba Found. Symp. 32), Elsevier/Excerpta Medica/North Holland, Amsterdam and New York, 1975, p.275.
—— *Size at Birth.* (Ciba Found. Symp. 27), Elsevier/Excerpta Medica/North Holland, Amsterdam and New York, 1974, p.418.
——*Human Rights in Health.* (Ciba Found. Symp. 23), Elsevier/Excerpta Medica/North Holland, Amsterdam and New York, 1974, p.311.
—— *Lipids, Malnutrition and the Developing Brain.* (Ciba Found. Symp. 3), Elsevier/Excerpta Medica/North Holland, Amsterdam and New York, 1972, p.337.
Fendall, N.R.E. *Auxiliaries in Health Care.* The Johns Hopkins Press, Baltimore and London, 1972.
Fox, T.F. 'The Greater Medical Profession'. *The Lancet,* Vol.II, 1956, pp.779-80.
Haldane, J.B.S. *Possible Worlds and Other Essays.* Chatto & Windus, London, 1927, pp.18-26.
Haraldson, S.R.S. 'Evaluation of Alaska Native Health Services'. *Alaska Medicine,* Vol.16, No.3, 1974.
Porter, Ruth and FitzSimons, D.W. (eds.) *Health Care in a Changing Setting: The UK Experience.* (Ciba Found. Symp. 43), Elsevier/Excerpta Medica/North Holland, Amsterdam and New York, 1976, p.188.
Wolstenholme, G.E. and O'Connor, Maeve (eds.) *Health of Mankind.* (Ciba Found. Symp.), Churchill Livingstone, Edinburgh, 1967, p.297.
Heller, Thomas. 'The Patterns of Medical Practice in England and the Third World'. *Contact*, No.33, p.10, Christian Medical Commission of World Council of Churches, Geneva, 1976.
Horn, J.S. *Away with All Pests.* Paul Hamlyn, London, 1969.
Illich, I. *Medical Nemesis – The Expropriation of Health.* Calder & Boyars, London, 1974.
—— *Limits to Medicine: Medical Nemesis – The Expropriation of Health.* Marion Boyars, London, 1976.
King, Maurice. *Medical Care in Developing Countries.* Oxford University Press, 1966.
Klein, Rudolf. 'Medical Manpower: 1 – How Much can Ancillaries Take Over?'. *British Medical Journal,* Vol.1, No. 6000, 1976, pp.25-30.
Leaper, D.J., *et al.* 'Computer-assisted Diagnosis of Abdominal Pain Using "Estimates" Provided by Clinicians'. *British Medical Journal,* No.11, 1972.
McKeown, Thomas. *The Role of Medicine: Dream, Mirage or Nemesis.* The Nuffield Provincial Hospitals Trust, London, 1976, p.180.
Mahler, H. 'Health – A Demystification of Medical Technology' in British Postgraduate Medical Federation Scientific Basis of Medicine series. *The Lancet,* 1975, pp.829-33.
Medical Alliance (1973) Editorial and Series *The Lancet* (beginning 5 May).
US Department of Health, Education and Welfare. *Medicine and Public Health in the People's Republic of China,* 1973.
Milio, Nancy M. *The Care of Health in Communities: Access for Outcasts.* MacMillan, New York, 1975, p.402.
Moore, M.F., *et al.* 'First-contact Decisions in General Practice: A Comparison between a Nurse and Three General Practitioners'. *The Lancet,* 14 April 1973.
Morley, D. *Paediatric Priorities in the Developing World.* Butterworths, London, 1973.
Myers, N. 'Of All Things People are the Most Precious'. *New Scientist* 65 No.931, 1975, pp.56-9.
Newell, K.W. (ed.) *Health by the People.* World Health Organisation, Geneva, 1975,

p.206.

Pellegrino, E.D. 'Future Interrelationships Among the Doctor, the Hospital and the Community: The Place for Advanced Technology and the Team Approach' in Proc. of International Conference on *Priorities for the Use of Resources in Medicine*. Fogarty International Center, Bethesda, Maryland, 1976.

People's Health Centre at Gonoshasthya Kendra, Nayarhat, District Dacca, Bangladesh. Quarterly newsletters.

Pitcairn, D.M. and Flahault, D. *The Medical Assistant – An Intermediate Level of Health Care Personnel*. Public Health Paper No.60, World Health Organisation, Geneva, 1974.

Rifkin, S. and Kaplinsky, R. *Health Strategy and Development Planning: Lessons from the People's Republic of China*. TALC (Teaching Aids at Low Cost reprint. Institute of Child Health, London, 1973.

Sadler, A.M., Sadler, B.L. and Bliss, A.A. *The Physician's Assistant – Today and Tomorrow*. Yale University Press, New Haven, Connecticut, 1972.

Schumacher, E.F. *Small is Beautiful: A Study of Economics as if People Mattered*. Blond & Briggs, London, 1973.

—— *People's Power*. National Council of Social Service, London, 1974.

—— *A Guide for the Perplexed*. Jonathan Cape, London, 1977.

Sidel, V.W. *Serve the People*. Josiah Macy Foundation, 1974.

—— 'Quality for Whom? Effects of Professional Responsibility for Quality of Health Care on Equity' in Proc. 1975 Annual Health Conference of the New York Academy of Medicine – The Professional Responsibility for Quality of Health Care: Long-Term Implications and Effects. *Bulletin of the NY Academy of Medicine*, 1975, p.21.

Sigerist, H.E. *Medicine and Human Welfare*. Yale University Press, New Haven, Connecticut. Reprinted by Consortium Press, Gaithersburg, Maryland, 1941.

Sox, H.C., *et al.* 'The Training of Physicians' Assistants: The Use of a Clinical Algorithm System for Patient Care, Audit of Performance and Education'. *New England Journal of Medicine*, 19 April 1973.

Wolstenholme, G.E. and O'Connor, Maeve (eds.) *Teamwork for World Health*. (Ciba Found. Symp.), Churchill Livingstone, Edinburgh, 1970, p.242.

*The Future of Schools of Allied Health: Helping Schools of Allied Health Maintain Their Viability* (A report on an Institute sponsored by the School of Health Studies, The University of New Hampshire, Durham, New Hampshire). American Society of Allied Health Professions, 1974, p.55.

'The Introduction of Satellites into Education Systems'. *Proc. R. Soc.,* London, September 1974.

Tichy, Monique K. (ed.) *Health Care Teams: An Annotated Bibliography*. Praeger Publishers, New York, 1974, p.177.

Weed, L.L. *Medical Records, Medical Education and Patient Care: The Problem Oriented Record as a Basic Tool*. Cleveland Press of Case Western Reserve University, Cleveland, Ohio, 1970.

# 2  DIVISION OF LABOUR: ROLES, RESPONSIBILITIES AND ACCOUNTABILITY WITHIN THE TEAM CONCEPT

Muriel Skeet

If I were asked to compose an epitaph on medicine throughout the twentieth century, it would read: brilliant in its discoveries, superb in its technological breakthroughs, but woefully inept in its applications to those most in need. Medicine will be judged not on its vast and rapid accumulation of knowledge *per se,* but on its trusteeship of that knowledge. We are now experienced and all that remains is the problem of translating what is common knowledge and routine medicine, and hence practice, to the other two-thirds of the world. The implementation gap must be closed.[1]

Turning from the wider international theme of health auxiliaries to nursing and its own substructures, we find in the European context four types of health care delivery: (i) the state system in the socialist countries; (ii) a nationalised health service in the UK; (iii) semi-nationalised services in the Scandinavian countries, particularly in Sweden; (iv) a system denominated by social insurance institutions and characterised by a more or less complete split between preventive and curative services, in central and southern Europe.

## The Nurse in the Team

Because the development of the nurse's role in recent years has been in direct response to demand and not on a planned basis, it is my belief that it now requires study to establish guidelines for forward planning. The function of the nurse must be determined by the needs of the patient, not by the presence or absence of other health professionals, nor by what other professionals do or do not wish to do themselves. But in the past decade or so we have decided that many of our traditional tasks, such as seeing that a patient eats enough of the right kind of food or has clean sheets on his bed, are non-nursing duties. We have decided that we can gain status by taking over routine technological procedures from physicians and we have taught that emotional involvement in our work is wrong. In fact, instead of extending our role in the field of nursing care, we have mutilated it.

27

The focus today is on keeping people well and outside hospital. With this emphasis the nurse is often the main health counsellor for the family and, in this role, shares with others the planning and giving of care. With this extended role thrust upon them and without adequate supporting services, nurses can be exploited and — even more serious — patients put at risk. I would suggest that in the United Kingdom the expanded role of the nurse has brought with it an even greater need for good back-up services — amongst which I would include that provided by nursing auxiliaries. Any auxiliary worker programme can only be as good as its own back-up services and as good as its supervision. Whilst I accept the view that every skilled worker has a responsibility and a necessity to teach those who are less skilled, I believe that in the nurse's case there is an urgent need to get her own educational system in good working order.

The trained nurse today is not a finished product — unlike her counterpart of thirty years ago. A certificate or diploma or degree simply means that certain requirements have been fulfilled which will give the holder the opportunity to follow a chosen career. To fit her for her extended role, the nurse will need continuing education in the form of in-service education, workshops, seminars and conferences, as well as independent study. Education and training are the subjects of other chapters, but I believe that in the UK our first priority must be urgent and radical action concerning our present nursing educational system. But we should also bear in mind, I believe, the words of a fellow-countrywoman, which are as apt today as they were a hundred years ago when they were written.

> It is quite surprising how many men, (and women do it too), practically behave as if the scientific end were the only one in view, or as if the sick body were but a reservoir for stowing medicines into, and the surgical disease only a curious case the sufferer has made for the attendant's special information.[2]

Again,

> A District Nurse must be of a yet higher class and of a yet fuller training than a hospital nurse, because she has no hospital appliances at hand at all and because she has to take notes of the case for the doctor who has no-one but her to report. . .[3]

The writer goes on to say, 'the love that springs from the sympathy of a close and accurate knowledge of the ways, habits, the lives of the poor is not a mere sentiment, but an active and fruitful enthusiasm.'[4] And lastly, 'Nursing must be treated like an Art in its relation to Medicine, Surgery and Hygiene: it is almost *co-extensive* with them.'[5] I am sure I have no need to name that wise and prophetic woman.

In developing countries the evolving role of nurses takes on a different dimension – that of evaluating community health needs, planning programmes, and recruiting, teaching and supervising health auxiliaries to provide direct health care as *alternatives* to themselves. It seems to me that we have confused the two possible roles of an auxiliary as defined by Fendall.[6] The auxiliary's role can be that of an *assistant to the professional,* working in a purely subordinate role or a *substitute for the professional,* carrying out her functions with a minimum of supervision and advice. For this workshop the definition has been very clearly stated. I believe that for the industrialised countries, such as the UK, it is the former role which is both suitable and acceptable.

## The Patient in the Team

Of course the nurse and the nursing auxiliary are not the only people who provide nursing care, and are not, therefore, our only consideration when we discuss the division of labour in nursing. There is the patient himself, there are his family and his friends and there are those other members of the community, volunteers.

I believe that the pyramid view of professionals in the health team must give way to the pie concept. Each member of the team is a wedge of different size according to the problem of the patient or the community, at a given time. In some situations a professional member of the team may have no part in the pie, but always – and there is no exception whatsoever – the patient and his family have a wedge. And that goes for every team – teams for cardiac surgery, for renal dialysis, for resuscitation and for laboratory and other procedures which have become part of medical routine, as well as for the primary health care team.

In the first place, health care is the responsibility, not of any member of the health professions, but of the individual. This makes a strong case for regarding as the linchpin of any health service the person with whom the individual first comes into contact when seeking medical help. In so-called advanced countries, this is often the doctor. For most of the world's people that contact is (or should be), someone known as the community health worker or health auxiliary, barefoot doctor, feldscher or whatever. As Monica Baly has reported,

> many patients who need care today are victims of their own behaviour:
> the drunken driver in the car crash; the heavy smoker with a
> carcinoma; the young man hooked on heroin; the girl with a septic
> abortion or the jet-happy executive with coronary heart disease.[7]

The need for the practice of preventive medicine is as great in the West
as it is in the Third World, and is 'Everybody's Business', as the recent
DHSS publication[8] pointed out.

Turning to the curative or therapeutic side, Virginia Henderson, in
her definition of the *unique* function of the nurse, describes the role, or
the wedge in the pie, of the patient. She defines the nurse's function as
being 'to assist the individual, sick or well, in the performance of those
activities contributing to health or its recovery (or to a peaceful death),
that he would perform unaided if he had the necessary strength, will, or
knowledge'. She goes on to say,

> *It is likewise her function to help the individual gain independence
> as rapidly as possible.* This aspect of her work, this part of her
> function, she initiates and controls: of this she is master. In addition
> (or as part of this defined function if it is broadly interpreted), she
> helps the patient to carry out the therapeutic plan as initiated by his
> physician. If the patient does not understand, accept and *participate*
> in his programme of care, the effort of the medical team is largely
> wasted. The sooner the person can care for himself, even carry out
> his own treatments, the better off he is.[9]

In the acute phase of an illness, the patient often wants decisions made
for him. But at other times he should be involved in all decision-making
— even whether he wishes to go or stay in hospital for his treatment.

## Community Participation

Many health education and care delivery systems have failed because they
have not made services both available and accessible to the people who need
them most. 'Good for the many' rather than 'best for the few' is now
becoming the byword in health services, as nations consider relative merits
of out-patient versus in-patient care; health centres versus hospitals;
preventive medicine versus curative medicine; and lower- and middle-level
trained health workers versus physicians and nurses. Rising costs are also
leading more and more countries to seek alternative models of health care

delivery.[10] Nurses led the way in developing non-professional personnel and others are following. It is because doctors have decided that they too need help that we are facing a crisis in nursing. Who is to be his assistant? Does he train another grade of medical worker or does he hand over routine tasks to the nurse? But certainly the rapid rise in the cost of health services is a critical problem facing both rich and poor countries.

> Within a few years several countries are likely to spend one tenth of their total resources on health care. But despite this vast expenditure, excessive and unnecessary services are provided for some, while important health needs of others go unmet.[11]

How is it possible to provide the right services at the right price and at the right time? How is it possible to get value for money in the health services? How many patients are worse off from being given the wrong treatment or no treatment and with what consequences? How much 'better' a service could have been provided within the resources locally available, by a higher trained person? The quality of service provided by all auxiliaries of limited education and training can, and should, be evaluated.

Whereas different countries have used a variety of innovative health approaches in their primary health care programmes, all of them have recognised that an untapped reservoir of human resources exists from which a body of primary health workers can be drawn and trained more rapidly, less expensively and in far greater numbers than doctors or nurses can be trained.[12] Full-time or part-time community health aides can be recruited from among villagers and can be trained in, or near, their own villages, so that they truly belong to the people they serve. But long before most people, Florence Nightingale recognised this: 'A people cannot really be helped except through itself'. . .'A people is its own soil and water. Others may plant, but it must *grow* its own produce.'[13]

In an increasing number of developing countries, the role of auxiliary health aides as members of the health care team has been recognised, not only as an important link between patients and the caring professionals in times of illness, but also as an easier means of communication between the people and health educators.[14] The auxiliary worker drawn from the community has advantages over the doctor or nursing student drawn from another area and isolated from the habits of speech and behaviour of rural people by years of education in an urban setting. The auxiliary worker should be in a better position to understand the real meaning of what is said to him by the patient and to find out what other remedies he may be taking and rituals or superstitions he may be observing, in response to the traditional medicine and culture of the community. And in this context we should not forget the practitioners of traditional medicine who provide the *only* source of health care for some four-fifths of the people in the developing countries. Acknowledging this reality, the World Health Organisation recently launched a programme in this field. Staff will collect and analyse information about what is being done, by whom and with what degree of success. Then training courses will be developed so that traditional practitioners can do better work in their communities and work in closer co-operation with the 'official' health service. Moreover the auxiliary is likely to stay in the community and thus provide continuity of care. Continuous service from an auxiliary with limited training may be better than service from a constantly changing succession of discontented young, and relatively inexperienced, doctors required to serve two years' rural posting before getting on with what they see as their ultimate career – hospital medicine or urban private practice.

### The Patient's Family in the Team

It is known that 96 per cent of nursing in the UK is undertaken by non-trained personnel. Giving the Nursing Lecture at a recent Annual General Meeting of the Royal College of Nursing, Professor Jean McFarlane said, 'Most nursing in society is carried out within the family by non-professionals, relatives and friends.' She went on to say,

> Only slowly are we learning that care is given by a team of professionals, all of whom have a contribution to make to decisions about care and methods of care. But that team also includes the patient and his lay-helpers who also make decisions about care and methods of care. The team must, therefore, assess together the needs and problems involved in caring for an individual and together reach decisions about their optimum solutions and the contribution best made by different members of that team.[15]

Peggy Nuttall recently stated, 'Never forget that we live in a do-it-yourself age. Nursing one single individual is not an especially difficult task.'[16] It is not – if you know how. Lucky indeed if you are a 'born nurse', but there are remarkably few in the world. I hesitate to quote Florence Nightingale again but she has already said it: 'It has been said and written scores of times that every woman makes a good nurse. I believe to the contrary that the very elements of nursing are all but unknown.'[17]

Some three years ago, I set up a study into the role and preparation of volunteers working within the reorganised NHS. For some time it had been apparent that the increased use of volunteers in the health and social services had brought problems as well as the much quoted 'extra dimension to patient care'. We hoped to achieve:

(i) Revision of the preparation of volunteers in order to meet the needs of patients and their families and to provide competent help to professionals.

(ii) Involvement of doctors, nurses and volunteers in a study which would: (a) make them more acutely aware of the needs of patients; (b) enable them to help their colleagues in other parts of the country to appreciate their patients' needs; and (c) enable them to take action to help in the preparation of volunteers to meet them.

The project was seen as an exploratory study, looking at a range of situations covering as many different Health Service activities and types of patients as possible. At the same time the patients' contacts and experience with voluntary help were examined. It was whilst I was analysing data for the interim report of this study that I was struck by the amount of nursing care the families of patients were giving and by the descriptions of their frustrations and needs. Those of you who have read *Life Before Death*[18] will know the kind of caring which is being given by families, often week after week and month after month. It was patently clear that they needed to be taught how to do competently those tasks which they were already having to do. This applied to families and friends caring for disabled persons, sick children, old people or dying relations, as well as the families of patients recently discharged from hospital or awaiting admission to hospital. Because of this experience, the British Red Cross launched at the beginning of 1976 a national campaign called 'Nursing for the Family'. This was a series of four sessions — each of one-and-a-half hours — demonstrating to members of the public basic nursing care procedures: how to make someone comfortable in bed, how to feed a helpless patient, move a paralysed patient, and so on. We monitored the programme and from an evaluation undertaken six months later we learned that there were further needs: young fathers wanted to know about child development and caring for their sick children. We also tried to interest them in learning how to care for their wives after influenza or immediately after surgery, childbirth, etc., but without a great deal of success! We identified not only the large number of people who were already giving nursing care but also a large number who wanted knowledge on maintaining a healthy family. As a result of this evaluation we designed six variations on the original theme in an attempt to meet some of these needs.

It is not difficult to imagine the kind of patience required to care for such people day after day with no visible light at the end of the tunnel. No wonder the stress and strain builds up until a physical outlet has to be found. Unfortunately, that dinosaur, the maiden aunt, who used to provide a relief service in such circumstances, is almost extinct. I believe we must provide much more in the way of relief services for such families. Surely this is the kind of back-up service which many district nurses and health visitors would welcome.

## The Volunteer as Auxiliary Worker

Throughout the time we were organising the Red Cross national campaign to help the patient's family, the study on the role and preparation of the volunteer in the NHS was continuing.

David Owen has said, 'We are all believers in the immense value of voluntary effort.'[19] Alas, as a member of the staff of a Voluntary Aid Society I know that today that is not true. However I do agree with what he goes on to say:

> No nation whose wealth is earned in the competitive markets of the world, will ever be able to afford to spare more than a limited percentage of able people for a whole-time commitment to areas of activity such as social welfare. This is a fact of life we have to accept.[20]

This is one of the main reasons why the role of the volunteer is no longer a fringe issue, but is increasingly occupying the centre stage of future decision-making. Volunteers are potentially the largest untapped source of labour that we have available to us. The greatest single contribution that the voluntary movement can make is to provide more people, more hours and more activity. It is to be hoped that the distinction between the paid and the unpaid will become progressively obscured, but this will only be achieved if the distrust by the fully trained is replaced by respect for the partially trained.

What can these partially trained volunteers do? Unfortunately, it would be more accurate to ask what *could* they do? The study, as the report *Health Needs Help*[21] states, revealed that often there is an enormous investment of devotion and deplorable lack of return. It was made obvious to the research workers that greater co-ordination, collaboration, communication and co-operation were vitally needed, not only by the statutory and co-ordinating agencies but also between the voluntary agencies and the volunteers themselves. These findings proved to many of us that there is a need for the volunteer to be included in the health team. But if she is to become a member of that team, she must receive adequate preparation for the job. The report of the Panel on Primary Health Care Teams stated: 'The team, being composed of members from a number of complementary disciplines, it is essential to define the objective of all its members so that there is a clear definition of their roles.'[22] To learn a professional role, one goes through a specific educational programme designed to teach those skills and impart the knowledge essential to carrying out the work within the role. Training is also a means of introducing the newcomer to the expectations of the other members of the team and of providing the opportunity to identify with it. I believe that if they are to be accepted and if they are to get satisfaction from their work, this must apply also to nursing auxiliaries, paid or unpaid.

The study recorded *expressed* needs. We collated material on what people — patients, families and professionals — saw as needs, and also how they thought some of them could be met by people other than health professionals. It was reported, for instance, that volunteers could have helped in solving many of the pre-admission and discharge problems of hospital patients. Geriatric patients required help with washing, bathing, getting to the WC, dressing and undressing as well as with shopping and the preparation of meals. Patients from other specialties needed help with bathing, moving, and, in the case of women, with the work they had to do as soon as they returned home: help with the children, housework, shopping, laundry, gardening and so on. Others needed help in taking their medicines or with simple treatments such as the instillation of eye and ear drops or with the renewal of a dressing.

As far as help and visits in hospital wards were concerned, doctors and nurses said that the value of the volunteer was 'just having someone from the outside world who has time to talk'. A small proportion said that they thought that volunteers could help with feeding, dressing and moving patients, whilst many listed 'help with transport', either to day centres or to diversional therapy classes, etc. The research workers themselves thought that hospital staff often did not take the opportunity to teach members of the family how to carry out tasks for the patient which they would have to undertake when the patient was discharged. The relations of those who were drug- or machine-dependent were given instructions, but very few of the stoma patients, for instance, received from their families and friends the understanding and help which they needed on returning home. It would seem that this could be one way to ensure continuity of care and also be a task within the scope of the prepared auxiliary. Indeed one of the most important roles the volunteer might fill is that of strengthening the bridge between hospital and community, smoothing the difficulties which so often inevitably arise when a patient enters, or is discharged from hospital.

In this survey of 250 patients, 22 per cent of the long-stay hospital patients and 15 per cent of the short-stay patients needed help with dressing and undressing when they reached home and were not receiving it. Non-nursing duties? A person's clothing is an extension of his personality. Day and night are marked by a change of clothing. This normal cycle is broken if the old or disabled or weak person has to stay in garments meant for sleep. The art of helping paralysed or arthritic limbs into garments without causing pain needs to be taught, however.

Many people needed advice on the general care of old people who were living with them: how to keep them active and interested; how to prevent constipation; how to help them to bath; the kind of food to give them and the amount of exercise they should encourage them to take. Those looking after old people who were ill needed additional information on the care of pressure areas and care of the mouth; how to change a soiled undersheet; how to encourage coughing to be productive; how to cope with lack of continence and with insomnia. Surely the auxiliary could take on this educational role, again providing a back-up service for the nurse responsible for the over-all care of an old person and his family. Members of the primary health care team, *as it is composed at present,* cannot give this kind of help as often as it is needed. The provision of such a service requires organisation and it requires teaching preparation for the auxiliary.

### Training for the Nursing Auxiliary

There is no doubt that with more women seeking remunerative employment, fewer volunteers are coming forward to meet a regular commitment during normal working hours. I can see, therefore, the

nursing auxiliary in the community undertaking those tasks which
nursing and VAD members of the Voluntary Aid Societies used to do
and are still doing, but to a more limited extent. It would seem logical
that the training programme of the latter should be used for the
former. This was advocated by the Royal College of Nursing in their
evidence to the Briggs Committee[23] and has been further recommended[24]
by District Nursing Officers (Teaching), such as James Smith of the
Brent Health District, who has made use of our syllabus and training
manual.[25] In its evidence to the Royal Commission on the National
Health Service, the RCN urged that all personnel in the NHS should
be given training for the functions they are expected to perform. It
goes on to say that

> nursing auxiliaries should be provided with training on an
> in-service basis. The parameters for the duties of auxiliaries should
> be laid down, and adhered to, so that these members of the nursing
> team are not exploited in order that cuts in the budget can be
> met. The Royal College of Nursing and the Nursing Auxiliaries
> Association, through a Liaison Committee, have considered the
> 'training needs of auxiliaries' and have urged the Department of
> Health and Social Security to issue guidance on the subject.[26]

The Royal College of Nursing also stated that the number of
auxiliaries who are required to support trained nurses is the number
that should be employed. How do we arrive at that figure?

During the study of the volunteer we found both health and welfare
workers used that overworked phrase 'supportive help.' When we
asked them to be more specific they listed such services as visiting,
listening (as opposed to hearing), cheering up, encouraging,
stimulating the mind, etc. Does one need training for this kind of
work? The Aves Committee Report, 1969, stated that

> volunteers who will be involved in close personal relationships
> will need, above all, to know something of human relationships
> and behaviour. They may need help in understanding the feelings
> and the attitudes of clients and in realising that the relationship
> has to be one of *mutual* acceptance. They need to learn something
> of the arts of communication and establishing relationships, of how
> to give and receive information and respect confidences. It is
> important that they should be able to judge how far they can go
> in dealing with a difficult situation and when and where to turn

for advice and help.[27]

Nurses are, at the present time, turning attention to their own training needs as counsellors or listeners. Should we not also be thinking of the nursing auxiliary and her needs? So often she is the only confidant of the patient.

Whatever training the auxiliary has, I am certain it is essential that that training is given by the professionals with whom she is working. In promoting the developed role for the nurse we should bear in mind that whilst it may largely mean the taking on of tasks previously undertaken by a medical practitioner it also includes teaching responsibilities for auxiliary workers.

### Responsibility and Accountability

All higher education is facing an era of accountability and nursing is no exception. The extending role of the clinical nurse has caused some uncertainty about ethical and legal implications as well as training requirements. The recent DHSS Circular (HC(77)22)[28] on this subject aroused some strong feelings, and understandably so. I believe these implications are of paramount importance. The area of competence of each profession must be clearly defined and for us, as members of the European Economic Community facing reciprocity of qualifications, it is essential that this be so. In view of this, each individual should be personally accountable for any action within his area of competence. There should be little difficulty, in fact, in allocating accountability in the 'clinical' field in instances of either commission or omission. The latter is, however, more difficult when it occurs in the service field.[29]

The question of personal accountability will remain unaltered. Each doctor and each nurse is accountable to his patient, to his employer or employing agency and to himself. As colleagues of different disciplines, we are not, in theory, accountable to each other, but we should, I suggest, query and discuss each other's actions when necessary. Only peer-group assessment will show whether or not an individual is performing his duties well, adequately or inadequately, and only such a group will be able to have its recommendations accepted by those it represents. It is for this reason that accountability should always be to a peer group. No professional body of men or women enjoys the idea of direction of its activities by others, however well intentioned or well informed. Only nurses, I suggest, really understand the problems faced by other nurses, just as only doctors fully recognise the difficulties of diagnostic situations faced by other doctors. I believe that no doctor has the right to determine a nurse's duties and that a doctor employing a nurse contradicts the concept of partnership between the professions. So does the content of the DHSS Circular (HC(77)22).[30]

Ethical issues frequently involve conflicting values and in many individual cases ethical standards are not specified in sufficient clarity to allow for unauthorised decision-making. As knowledgeable participants in health care practice and research, professional nurses should involve themselves in institutional policy-making and review committee activities. Nurses must also be informed regarding the legal parameters affecting practitioner-patient relationships.[31] Salary should reflect the level of responsibility, experience and preparation of the recipient. Both legal status and methods of payment will affect the direction and the rate at which expansion of the role occurs.

## The Team Concept

In considering the work and training of the nursing auxiliary, I believe it is vital that we bear in mind that the team concept must include all those medical, nursing (including midwifery), paramedical and auxiliary professions involved in the diagnosis, care, rehabilitation and the welfare of the patient. The standards of expectation of the community have increased exponentially in our lifetime and there is no reason to believe that this growth of demand will not continue in the same way. Having accepted the concept, there are two main problems to be faced:

(i) to decide which services need to be offered and their ranking order of priority;
(ii) to recognise the individual capabilities of the various work groups and their availability in national terms.

The need has to be measured first. The total task of investigating and sometimes curing illness has to be quantified and then broken into constituent parts that can be allocated to the appropriate staff group having both the training to fill the role and the interest in doing so efficiently. There is nothing sacrosanct about the particular grades of health service manpower which have evolved. Indeed, as many of us here well know, such terms as doctor or dentist, as well as nurse, imply a homogeneity of job content within countries and between countries which simply does not exist.[32] I sometimes think that it would be better to do away with all existing grades, to begin anew with what the patient and his family need; allocate the constituent parts and then introduce new names for the workers who will provide, or help to provide, the care and therapy. The essential principle is that no patient should be treated by a person with greater skill or in facilities of greater sophistication than are needed to provide effective treatment. Dr Maurice King has stated this principle clearly.[33] We must also remember that team-work implies the sharing of responsibility, the delegation of it and the authority to carry out responsibilities and duties delegated. Characteristics of team-work include mutual trust and openness; that is, respect for and acknowledgement of each member's expertise both as a practitioner and as an individual. The question of leadership is raised only when this is absent.

## Notes

1. Alexander Dorozynski, *Doctors and Healers,* International Development Research Center (Ottawa, 1975).
2. W.J. Bishop and S. Goldie, *A Bio-bibliography of Florence Nightingale* (London, Dawson, 1962).
3. Ibid.
4. Ibid.
5. Ibid.
6. N.R.E. Fendall, *Auxiliaries in Health Care,* Publication for the Josiah Macy, Jr. Foundation by the Johns Hopkins Press (Baltimore and London, 1972).
7. Monica Baly, *Nursing and Social Change* (London, William Heinemann, 1975).
8. A Consultative Document: *Prevention and Health: Everybody's Business* (London, HMSO, 1976).
9. Virginia Henderson, *The Basic Principles of Nursing Care* (International Council of Nurses (ICN), 1969).
10. V. Djukanovic and E.P. Mach, *Alternative Approaches to Meeting Basic Health Needs in Developing Countries* (UNICEF/WHO, 1975).
11. B. Abel-Smith, *Value for Money in Health Services* (London, Heinemann, 1976).
12. Kenneth Newell (ed.), *Health by the People* (WHO, 1975).
13. W.J. Bishop and S. Goldie, op.cit.
14. Muriel Skeet, 'Some First Ports of Call', *Journal of Tropical Medicine and Hygiene* (January 1977).
15. J.K. McFarlane, Nursing Lecture, Annual General Meeting of the Royal College of Nursing of the United Kingdom (1975).
16. P.D. Nuttall, Battersea Memorial Lecture delivered to the Association of Integrated and Degree Courses in Nursing, London, 1975.
17. W.J. Bishop and S. Goldie, op.cit.
18. Ann Cartwright *et al., Life Before Death* (London, Routledge and Kegan Paul, 1970).
19. David Owen, *Politics and Medicine* (London, Heinemann, 1976).
20. David Owen, op.cit.
21. Muriel Skeet and E. Crout, *Health Needs Help* (London, Blackwell Scientific

Publications, 1977).
22. British Medical Association Board of Science Education, *Primary Health Care Team* (London, BMA, 1974).
23. Royal College of Nursing, *Evidence to the Committee on Nursing* (Briggs) (1972).
24. J.P. Smith, 'Training Nurse Auxiliaries', *Queen's Nursing Journal* (May 1976).
25. Joan Markham, *Nursing,* The Authorised Manual of the St John Ambulance Association and Brigade, St Andrew's Ambulance Association and British Red Cross Society (London, 1969).
26. Royal College of Nursing, *Evidence to the Royal Commission on the National Health Service, submitted by the RCN* (London, Royal College of Nursing of the UK, 1977).
27. G.M. Aves, *The Voluntary Worker in the Social Services* (London, Allen and Unwin, 1969).
28. DHSS, *Health Services Management: The Extending Role of the Clinical Nurse. Legal Implications and Training Requirements,* HC(77)22 (June 1977).
29. Royal Society of Medicine/Josiah Macy Foundation, *The Greater Medical Profession* (Josiah Macy Foundation, 1973).
30. DHSS Circular, *Health Services Management.*
31. Barbara Tate, *The Nurse's Dilemma* (International Council of Nurses and Florence Nightingale International Federation, 1977).
32. B. Abel-Smith, op.cit.
33. Maurice King, *Medical Care in Developing Countries* (London, Oxford University Press, 1966).

# 3 AUXILIARIES: WHO NEEDS THEM? A CASE STUDY IN NURSING

Melissa Hardie

**Objectives**

This policy study, which is not yet completed, is an attempt to fill some gaps in knowledge about the nursing auxiliary by providing information on three particular policy aspects of nursing auxiliary usage:

(i) employment and deployment;
(ii) current and planned instruction programmes;
(iii) work patterns and job descriptions.

It is under these headings that I will draw out some of the findings.

The working definition of auxiliaries which was used for the purpose of this work is the following;

> a person working within the nursing establishment managed by nursing officers, who has less than or no recognised UK nursing qualification, and who is not a student nurse, pupil nurse, or pupil midwife.

This is generally based upon the Nurses and Midwives Whitley Council definition, and equates in definition to Level III nursing personnel as designated by the International Council of Nurses.[1]

Specifically excluded in this initial project was the nursing auxiliary or aide as employed in the mental health services, though it is hoped to carry out a subsequent companion study in this field.

**Resources**

The Scottish Home and Health Department and the Department of Health and Social Security agreed jointly to fund our work for a two-year period (1976-7). Miss Hockey was appointed grant-holder and supervisor to the study, with myself as research officer. In addition to secretarial assistance, we have had access to all Edinburgh University computer and back-up services. The Nursing Research Unit's statistical and computer adviser has collaborated in the work from the initial stages. An experienced nurse researcher helped us with coding, and a registered nurse tutor with the analysis of training programmes. A small advisory panel, representing government, service and academic interests, was formed to comment on progress and direction of the study, and an interim report was submitted to them and to government departments in January 1977. The final report is to be submitted in January 1978. A further proposal, based upon subject-areas emerging from our policy analysis, has been submitted for funding.

## Methods

The methods employed in this project have been the postal questionnaire, document analysis and the semi-standardised interview. Following an initial pilot study in one English region, every regional, area, and district nursing officer and equivalent in the United Kingdom was invited to participate. The pilot response rate of slightly over 95 per cent led us to believe that the subject under investigation is of great interest to nursing administrators. As a means of eliciting factual policy information over the widest geographical spread, we were satisfied that the postal questionnaire was the most efficient and economical in cost and time for the respondents. In summary, the regional return was 100 per cent, the area return of 102 replies represented 91 per cent and the 235 district replies, including post-graduate teaching hospitals, equalled 87 per cent. This produced an overall 88.6 per cent return in the general study phase.

Different questionnaires were used for regional and area nursing officers on the one hand, and for district nursing officers on the other. Regional and area nursing administrators were asked about four main topics:

(i) sources of information for planning and monitoring; (ii) normal channels of communication; (iii) special discussions and studies in progress; (iv) opinions on the suitability of current information for manpower planning.

District nursing officers who are at operational level were asked, first, for factual details covering all aspects of nursing auxiliary employment and instruction and, second, for opinions about information requirements and the appropriateness of auxiliaries in patient care. Third, they were asked for such relevant documentation as was available.

The second method therefore has been document analysis — the study of the contents of job descriptions, training schedules, lists of duties allowed and lists of duties not allowed to nursing auxiliaries. The third method involved the interviewing of a small number of nursing auxiliaries in three locations, exploratory to future possible work.

**Employment and Deployment**

Based upon 1975 government statistics, and by masking all geographical and speciality distribution of nurses, we obtain the figures shown in Table 3.1. If these gross statistics are set against various regional and

Table 3.1: Nursing Manpower Summary — Great Britain
(All Nursing and Midwifery Staff), 1975

| Staff | Number | Percentage of Total, Including Learners | Percentage of Total, Not Including Learners |
|---|---|---|---|
| Qualified nurses and midwives | 202,464 | 49.8 | 66.1 |
| Student and pupil nurses, midwifery students and nursing cadets | 99,673 | 24.5 | |
| Other nursing and midwifery staff (i.e. auxiliaries) | 103,679 | 25.5 | 33.9 |

Source: DHSS, *Health and Personal Social Services Statistics for England*, with summary tables for Great Britain, 1976.

national suggestions for appropriate ratios, of which six different sets appeared in our data, immediate questions are raised about the popular notions of balance and imbalance of nursing staff, and the desirable ratio between auxiliary and qualified staff. (Table 3.2)

Other nursing administrators suggested that in no environment should auxiliaries constitute more than 20, 25 or $33\frac{1}{3}$ per cent of the nursing work-force.

In summarising this picture in another way, it may be said that in staffing situations where students or learners are employed, the suggestions are that 1 in 3, 1 in 4, or 1 in 5 of staff may be an auxiliary. Where no learners are used for staffing, 1 in 2, 1 in $2\frac{1}{5}$ and 1 in 3 may be an auxiliary. With these being very wide differences indeed, one must ask upon whose needs these suggestions are based?

In fact, total employment figures conceal wide differences between

Table 3.2: Suggested Ratios of Nursing Staff, Produced by
Respondents as Result of National and Regional Guidance Memoranda

| | Training Hospitals within Districts (percentage) | | | Non-training Hospitals (percentage) | | |
|---|---|---|---|---|---|---|
| Levels I and II (SRN and SEN) | 40 | 40 | $33\frac{1}{3}$ | $66\frac{2}{3}$ | 60 | 50 |
| Learners | 40 | 38 | $33\frac{1}{3}$ | | | |
| Auxiliaries | 20 | 22 | $33\frac{1}{3}$ | $33\frac{1}{3}$ | 40 | 50 |

districts. Our findings show that the proportion of auxiliaries in the
hospital service ranged from 4 to 63 per cent of total nursing staff, and
in the community services from 0 to 34 per cent. Eighteen community
divisions do not employ auxiliaries at all, though there is no hospital
division in our study which is without auxiliaries. The most usual
proportion of auxiliary employment was between $33\frac{1}{3}$ and 50 per cent
of total nursing staff, excluding learners. Only one district employed
5 per cent or less, whereas fourteen districts employed 50 per cent or
more.

Within districts there is also variation between different divisions,
units and wards, though we do not have sufficient detail to be able
to discern patterns in this. Some further light on policies which affect
deployment, however, appears in the section on working patterns.

At present we have no objective means of estimating whether
qualified first- and second-level (state registered and state enrolled)
nurses could entirely staff our health services, even if money were
available. Against this assertion, however, must be considered the
vast discrepancy between the numbers of nurses on the Register and
the Roll, and those actually employed. As one example of this
difference, the General Nursing Council for England and Wales
reported in 1976[2] that only 25-30 per cent of nurses on the Register
and the Roll were practising as nurses. Of the remainder, 10 per cent
were known to be over statutory retirement age, 25 per cent of
mailing addresses were known to be out of date and untraceable, and
an unknown quantity could be dead. In that year 18,000 new
state registered nurses (3 years' training) and 11,500 new state
enrolled nurses (2 years' training) were added to the Register and the
Roll respectively. At this rate of qualification, English and Welsh
nurses alone could in four years replace currently employed auxiliaries,
assuming that all of the qualified wished to work. This ignores the
pool of the estimated 60 per cent of already qualified nurses, who for

any number of reasons are not now working as nurses, in Scotland, Northern Ireland, England and Wales.

Though we have heard increasingly about the difficulties of newly qualified nurses obtaining employment over the past three years, we have no figures to support it. The situation was totally the reverse from previous years, when we could not find enough nurses. We must ask whether it is difficulties with such institutional barriers as part-time/full-time work, tight economy, the unattractiveness of working conditions or the level and nature of the work which keep the qualified away, but nevertheless sustain a high level of auxiliary usage. Auxiliaries are filling a need which the qualified do not fill, despite an expensive training, but we do not know why. In our discussions it would be useful to us to know of international attempts that may have been made to ensure that staff actually trained by the system are fully utilised before others are employed to take over some or all of their work.

Several nursing administrators indicated that the highest use of auxiliaries was in geriatric wards, divisions, and other chronic illness environments. They also indicated that without auxiliaries they would not be able adequately to staff wards at night or at weekends. If we then consider that 50 per cent of National Health Service beds are occupied by people over 65 years of age, who in terms of nurse dependency are heavy users, and because of their disablements and length of stay require night and weekend help consistently, further questions arise. We must ask whether we need nurses or auxiliaries? On what basis are we making decisions about ratios: on the basis of the needs of patients, or because of maldistribution and malpreparation of staff, or upon the professional fears of qualified nurses? Because of the astonishing variation in use of auxiliaries between districts, can we lend credence to the theory that our planning mechanisms are in any way meeting patient and nursing needs, if they are based on notional ratios which are seldom met in practice? What are the ramifications for training programmes, at all levels, even if ratios are seen to meet patient needs?.

## Current and Planned Instruction Programmes

A recent American study indicated that 60 per cent of nursing work was carried out by any nursing workers from the auxiliary to the qualified.[3] Twenty-eight per cent was somewhat more complex and should be allocated only to nurses trained to Levels I or II. Twelve per cent would require a fully qualified nurse. British studies have made estimates of this as well, and the use of some current patient-dependency indices can result in such estimates. Based on sixty training programmes for auxiliaries that we have investigated, the interchangeability of instruction and resulting duties could be seen to be almost complete. All task areas covered in the registered nurse syllabus of the General Nursing Council, with the exception of injections and certain forms of drainage, are being carried out somewhere in the UK by auxiliaries. This does not, of course, mean that every auxiliary is carrying out the whole spectrum of nursing duties on a regular basis. Nevertheless, in most health care settings, one could make this statement about Level I and II nurses as well.

This finding in itself may not be so surprising, because in the words of one nursing administrator, 'almost any worker with instruction and supervision can be taught to carry out any procedure or group of related procedures.' It only becomes startling when one finds that training resources as well as continued instruction and support facilities are disparate in the extreme. In 1971, the survey which was carried out for the Committee on Nursing (the Briggs Committee),[4] on the training for auxiliaries and assistants, found that in over 50 per cent of hospitals no training at all, induction or later instruction, was offered to these workers. One-half of the auxiliaries in their representative sample agreed that they had received no training at all.

Our data show that orientation days and in-service training in some form or another are currently offered by about 70 per cent of districts, but time devoted to it is only partially quantifiable. It is also notable here that approximately one-third of the thirty pilot interviews we carried out with nursing auxiliaries revealed that even though the hospitals concerned did offer some auxiliary instruction on a formal basis, the individual being interviewed had not received the training for one reason or another.

Thirteen districts only (6 per cent) stated that they offered no instruction, 26 districts (11 per cent) reported offering a formal course of instruction covering 2 weeks or more. We have a large amount of data on hours and days of instruction which is being prepared for the final report. However, it is particularly interesting to note that in only 31 per cent of districts is the instruction offered under the auspices of the nurse educational system, even though all of the workers are managed by nurse managers. In only 13 per cent of districts is there a clinical instructor normally available to help auxiliaries to learn.

These few facts may support the dismay that some administrators

(10 per cent) displayed towards the use of the word 'nursing' as applied to auxiliaries, and of course related to the now common issue of what are and are not nursing duties. However, the training programmes mentioned above, which attempt perhaps to produce a 'mini-nurse' in 0 to 14 days, supported by elements of over 200 job descriptions that we received, cannot help but raise the question as to how realistic these nursing administrators are? There can be no doubt, despite the bias in documentation towards routines, special tasks and domestic duties, that auxiliaries are *nursing*. From the interviews with auxiliaries themselves, there is also no doubt that they are nursing patients in addition to looking after the equipment which aid patients and nurses.

Because of ward assignment policies and other factors such as age and permanent local residence, auxiliaries are more likely to be a very stable element in the nursing team. This was acknowledged by nursing administrators and by auxiliaries themselves, both as a source of support to the head nurses and student nurses, and as a source of conflict. The head nurse, over time, has knowledge of the responsibilities that a particular nursing auxiliary can undertake and may rely heavily on her. Student nurses, especially in the first week or two in a new environment, may be taught their duties and procedures by the auxiliary. Nevertheless, the teaching and institutional customs demand that, regardless of ability or the recognised role of an auxiliary as a teacher herself, the auxiliary remains at the bottom of the hierarchy and can foresee no change. While this may suit some workers because of home and social conditions, our interviews revealed a strong consciousness of the static career situation and the limitations of their working situation, and extreme reluctance in accepting it. The training needs of auxiliaries are viewed as a lower priority than those of nurse learners, at the same time as it is acknowledged that their stability may enable the environment to continue to function.

A common charge is made that nursing standards are falling. If standards are inculcated by education and training, and persons nursing patients are not in fact being instructed to them, what is one measuring in trying to measure standards: the standards of care, or the level of ignorance? If one hypothesises that auxiliaries in making up 25 per cent of total nursing manpower, provide even 25 per cent of nursing care to patients, then it might be feasible to allocate 25 per cent of training resources towards their needs. On any formal basis this is not being done. The assumption must be that

administrators and nurses generally believe that familiarity with the
particular routine of a ward or community duty will ensure
safe and adequate nursing care of patients. Or are we again viewing
the training needs of a work-force based upon what the nursing
system has left over? If, as Miss Hockey asserts in a recent paper,
the nurse's task is to assess the total patient needs and make
appropriate arrangements for these needs to be met,[5] how are these
seen and judged to be appropriate arrangements? The third section
will raise similar questions.

## Working Patterns and Job Descriptions

Significantly linked to the mention of ratios is the constant mention
of 'supervision'. 'Adequate supervision', seldom defined in any way
within the replies, is seen as the quality of nursing behaviour which
legitimates the use of auxiliaries within the system. In the key word
analysis employed in the study, it was the single most common word
concept appearing in opinion statements. In few cases were auxiliaries
objected to in principle or considered as incapable of delivering care;
if supervised, then auxiliaries were invaluable, even essential, and in
some cases valued above qualified nurses for eagerness to please,
kindness to patients, as well as for the ability to make a little time for
the patient's smaller needs. In this vein, the auxiliary is seen as the
patient's friend and the nurse's agent.

One cannot help being amused at the irony of the following
comment: 'We find auxiliaries essential to our nursing service. If this
member of staff was reduced, additional learners and trained staff
would have to be employed.' Herein the auxiliary is the *nurse,* and
the basis for calculating the remainder of the staff. Throughout the
replies there was little or no reference to any change of working
patterns due to the employment of auxiliaries in greater or lesser
number; the danger points were rather seen to be in the functioning
relationship between supervisor and varying levels or ratios of
auxiliaries, not in the sophistication or simplicity of the work which
was to be carried out.

Other comments described the auxiliary as the 'front-line nurse',
the 'backline of the nursing service', the 'core' and the 'base', in
addition to being the 'anchor' in certain environments while learners
and qualified staff moved in and out. On a five-point positive-
negative scale, opinions of nursing administrators are strongly positive
to the use of auxiliaries. The appeal to *supervision* must be seen,
however, against local employment ratios before it is taken as a positive

work pattern. The major trade-off in nursing employment appears to be between the fully trained nurse and the auxiliary. Where there are few registered nurses, there are many nursing auxiliaries and vice versa. The implications in this inverse ratio for the ability to supervise, depending upon its meaning, are obvious. We must ask about the definitions of this function of supervision: what does it mean?

Twenty-five per cent of districts identify wards or parts of health care facilities where as a matter of policy auxiliaries are not employed. Is this a starting-point for discussion of rationalising policy towards the use of auxiliary personnel? Intensive care units, coronary care units, special care units, operating theatres and venereal disease clinics are the most common among these, but certain districts also identify a wide variety of other types of environment, for which they may have technical or traditional reasons. Nevertheless, 75 per cent of districts, at least on paper, do not make these distinctions. Are we viewing working patterns based on the needs and wants of nurses, backed by their training, to work in more technical settings? Or is a case made for a generally trained auxiliary to carry out the same tasks in all environments?

Community health divisions employ far fewer auxiliaries. This may partly be tradition, and also partly be due to the fairly unclear definitions, or a feeling of insecurity about nursing supervisory obligations towards the untrained. Over 50 per cent of areas are discussing or have discussed a reorientation of auxiliary deployment, in regard to preparing them jointly for the hospital and the community, but no evaluation of a project such as this is known to us. Six districts and four areas are interested in the possibility of joint training for home helps and nursing auxiliaries. This may be a way in which auxiliaries are seen by nurses to meet their needs best, by allowing the nurses the practice of technical and organisational skills, for which they have trained so long. Nevertheless, one can surmise that there will be further difficulties with division of labour and appropriate instruction if greater numbers of more seriously ill patients are nursed at home.

Permeating our study is the need expressed by nurses to be everywhere at once. They believe they should be doing all the work at all levels to ensure safety to patients, a smooth organisation and a competent recognised profession. But, because nurses feel that they may not be meeting patient needs, they are concerned about their tools, which can be briefly listed as: professional standards, institutional barriers, manpower and information. The tendency, therefore, is to bemoan the high level of auxiliary employment — even if it is needed — rather than to ask specifically why they are needed and then to place priority on deciding about their appropriate use.

## Notes

1. World Health Organisation, Export Committee on Nursing, *Fifth Report* (1966).
2. General Nursing Council of England and Wales, *Annual Report* for the year 1975-6 (1976).
3. June B. Somers, 'Purpose and Performance: A System Analysis of Nurse Staffing', *Journal of Nursing Administration* (February 1977).
4. Social and Community Planning Research, *Briggs,* survey methodology and results, Working Papers, February 1971.
5. Lisbeth Hockey, 'The Nurse's contribution to care in a changing setting', *Journal of Advanced Nursing,* 2 (1977), pp.147-56.

# 4 NURSING AUXILIARIES – THE ECONOMIC ARGUMENT

Lisbeth Hockey

What is the economic argument? Most commonly it is a polite way of saying, 'We can't afford it.' We blame lack of money for many weaknesses in health care provision. Often lack of money is not the root cause at all, but blaming something outside our control provides a convenient escape from personal and professional responsibility.

I would like to take the economic argument just a little further, but not beyond the concern of health care professionals. Although the discipline and science of economics has developed its own body of knowledge, expertise and its own language, it is my firm belief that applied economics in the field of health care should be based on interdisciplinary team work, with nurses as members of that team.

The fundamental issues of economic theory are concerned with the inter-relationships between demand, supply and price or cost. Economic theory comes into its own at a time of scarcity, at a time when the demand for goods or services exceeds their supply. In the market-place the effect of excessive demand is a rise in price, a rise in the cost of the respective good or service to the consumer, which thereby normally reduces the demand and brings the price down again. Exceptions to this stabilising mechanism are those goods and services which are indispensable to the consumer, those for which there are no acceptable alternatives. For many of us, coffee and our motor car may be examples of such indispensables and the economist refers to a demand which remains unchanged in spite of a change in price as 'inelastic'.

Health care costing is not amenable to the market-place pattern of price stabilisation. The price mechanism cannot be used to reduce demand for health care as this itself would increase the health problems, thereby having the effect of increasing rather than decreasing the cost of care in the long term. Moreover, paradoxically, a measure of success in health care by overcoming major killers, infectious diseases and reducing infant mortality results inevitably in more protracted and complex problems associated with the survival of the unfit. A country with a National Health Service such as the UK is unable to make any substantial transfer of cost from the government to the consumer, although tax increases and selective payments for certain items are possible and have already been introduced.

Some public welfare services will not be demanded in excess of their utility even if they are free at the time of utilisation; the provision of water and collection of refuse are such examples. Any public service which does not appear to be self-limiting has to find some way to control expenditure. The health care system is not self-limiting mainly because of increased expectations by the consumers and advances in health care science which continue to increase the utility of intervention; thus an increasing number of conditions become amenable to treatment which sometimes is extremely costly. The health service in the UK has shown a drastic increase in cost since its inception and salaries of health workers represent a major item. Within the salary budget it is the salary of nurses which absorbs the highest cost, not because they are the best-paid workers but because they provide a round-the-clock service (Table 4.1). It is understandable, therefore, that this particular item should come under close scrutiny – one of the main reasons for the economic argument.

Clearly, it would be naïve simply to resort to the 'We can't afford it' escape. Patients need nursing and, if current trends continue, the need for nursing care is likely to increase rather than decrease. We therefore have to ask the question, 'How can good health care be provided at reasonable cost?' posed by Robert Maxwell[1] in his introduction to the McKinsey Report, entitled *Health Care – The Growing Dilemma,* in the hope that we can produce some sort of system which will give us value for money. In this context it is helpful to refer to Professor Abel-Smith who, in his book *Value for Money in the Health Services,*[2] cogently argues some of the dilemmas we are faced with against some possible solutions available to us. I use the term 'solutions' advisedly, because I do not side with those who almost seem to enjoy telling themselves and others that they can't do anything without money.

I consider that it is dangerous to talk oneself into such a state and that it is more often than not simply an excuse for inactivity and procrastination. At the same time, I recognise that the economic situation can cause some genuine frustration and that the temptation to opt out and give up is great. For those who persevere, the challenge of the recession can be as rewarding as any challenge. It stimulates initiative and imagination and encourages novel ideas, perhaps even a measure of entrepreneurship and risk-taking. I hope, therefore, that we can view the difficult financial era in a positive way, as giving us the

Table 4.1: Hospital and Specialist Services Salaries and Wages

| Hospital Service | 1965-6 | 1975-6 |
|---|---|---|
| Medical | 1,391 | 7,473 |
| Nursing | 23,820 | 127,289 |
| Medical auxiliary and dispensary | 2,381 | 13,087 |
| Hospital administrative and clerical | 1,892 | 10,932 |
| Domestic and catering | 10,625 | 55,552 |
| Tradesmen and others | 3,313 | 11,673 |
| Laboratory, etc., services and trading concerns | 2,346 | 16,400 |
| Laundry staff | 1,095 | 4,731 |
| Total | 46,863 | 247,137 |

Source: Scottish Health Statistics 1975; Information Services Division, Common Services Agency for the Scottish Health Service, Edinburgh, HMSO.

opportunity to, or perhaps forcing us to, reflect seriously on hitherto accepted conventions with their inherent comfortable security and to evaluate them in the light of changing needs and resources. In order to do this, we need to apply not only our common sense, our intelligence and our professional expertise, but also the less familiar but promising and exciting methods of economic analysis. It is for this reason that I stressed earlier the need for an interdisciplinary partnership. The fact that such new methods for the critical appraisal of our health care system are available is another important reason for engaging in the economic argument rather than sitting back in self-pity and despair, the seed-bed of the most infectious of all diseases, namely apathy, with its almost inevitable complications of low morale and loss of job satisfaction.

Because the demand, quite apart from the need, for health care exceeds the supply, health care which includes nursing is an economic good, a scarce resource which needs to be dispensed on some principles of priority allocation. The identification of priorities requires informed decision-making and it is in this area that analysis based on economic science can help. It adds another less emotive and subjective dimension to the process of resource allocation than that employed by ambitious medical specialists, protective nursing generalists and opposing party politicians. It is not a coincidence that welfare economics is a rapidly developing specialty. Applied health economics, as a branch of welfare economics, is an acknowledged growth area, not only in the UK but in most industrialised societies. It is epitomised by the increasing amount of literature on the subject, for example the works by Cooper and Culyer,[3] Cooper,[4] Culyer[5] and Price[6] and by the increasing number of health economists being employed by the government health departments. Here in Scotland, it is further demonstrated in the sponsorship by government of a Health Economics Research Unit in Aberdeen.

Basically, the function of health economists is to demonstrate the results of alternative patterns of health care and the two most commonly employed techniques are those of analyses of cost-benefit and cost-effectiveness.

As there is sometimes confusion between these two types of analysis, a brief explanation is called for.

Very broadly, the cost-benefit approach is an attempt to measure systematically projects or programmes in the public sector where no market price can be determined and where the provision and consumption of services within the project or programme has general, far-reaching and long-term implications. Three components are necessary for such an approach: first, all costs should be enumerated as fully as possible; second, all expected benefits should be enumerated as fully as possible; and, third, the time period over which both costs and benefits can be expected to accrue should be identified as far as possible and should be built into the cost-benefit equation. Short- and long-term benefits may have to be identified. My emphasis on 'as fully as possible' and 'as far as possible' is intended to convey the difficulty of the exercise with its considerable hypothetical component. In addition, there may be, indeed there are bound to be, value judgements in the identification of benefits. Thus, some people may consider the survival of severely handicapped people a benefit, whilst others may wish to place their desired benefit on the achievement of an acceptable quality of life rather than on its duration. Other choices of health-related goals remain. Health resources could be concentrated on the environment with the objective of minimising health risks. Thus, on the one hand, a society could spend its health resources on good buildings – schools, offices, factories – or on the provision of parks and open spaces, on clean air measures or on road safety and other similar efforts conducive to healthy living. On the other hand, a society could equally use its health resources for preventive care of individuals, such as health education, immunisation or screening. Alternatively, the bulk of health resources may be expended on diagnostic and therapeutic services, with the further conflict between issues such as expensive transplant surgery and good care for the long-term sick, the aged and the mentally retarded. The economist should not enter into the debate on the nature of benefits but should calculate the respective costs of different projects in relation to the benefits enumerated for him. Thus he will calculate, for example, the cost-benefit of a screening programme in the light of cost of treatment of undiagnosed disease and of loss of production through the illness or untimely death. The decision on whether the programme can be afforded or not will be taken by those who are charged with the responsibility of providing health care facilities. Such a decision will be aided by the objectively calculated figures provided by the economist.

Cost-effectiveness is a special and more restricted form of cost-benefit. It tends to be employed when the various benefits are difficult to measure or where the benefits thought to accrue from alternative schemes are so unlike that they cannot be set against each other and compared. In a cost-effectiveness approach, costs are calculated and compared for alternative ways of achieving a given agreed set of results. In this type of analysis the question of whether the result can be afforded does not rise, as it is taken for granted that the choice lies in the methods of achieving the results rather than in the results themselves; different patterns of nursing care could be an example.

Cost, as can be seen, enters into both types of analysis. The economist deals with many different types of cost and I believe that at least some of these have an application to health care in general and to the provision of nursing care in particular. Capital costs, recurrent costs, average cost, marginal cost, opportunity cost and consumer cost are examples, and I would like to enlarge a little on some of them. Capital and recurrent costs are household terms for all who are responsible for the preparation of budgets or whose work is directly related to a budget. Average cost: as far as average cost is concerned I appreciate that its meaning is well understood. What tends to be overlooked is the danger implicit in all averages, the cancelling out of extremes which may conceal important features. I consider that this is particularly important in the interpretation of average costs of an enterprise like the Health Service, with its many diverse and complex components. Although many components are itemised and costed separately, the problem of the average remains. Average cost of nurses' salaries can be cited as an example. It becomes easily apparent that salaries have a different costing value depending on the time of day and the day of the week, due to extra duty payments. Such differences get lost in the calculation of total and average costs, but they are important to the economic argument, and I believe that fluctuations in salary costs throughout days, weeks and months warrant much more careful examination.

Marginal cost: marginal cost appears to be a neglected concept in health care costing and I would recommend a closer study of its potential. Marginal cost is defined as the cost of providing an additional unit of whatever is being costed. Thus, it could be an additional hour of nursing time, an additional bed, an additional member of staff, an additional course within a training programme, an additional learner within the programme, etc. It is obvious that such an additional unit may result in an increase of average cost. It is possible, however, for the cost to remain constant, the additional unit being absorbed within existing resources. Sometimes the average or even the total cost can be reduced by the provision of an additional unit. This is particularly relevant when an enterprise is being costed which has an income related to the expenditure. The economic argument must include consideration of marginal cost and marginal benefit, that is the pay-off resulting from providing an additional unit.

Opportunity cost: opportunity cost refers to the value of alternatives which could have been chosen instead of the one which has incurred the specific cost – the cost of a forgone opportunity. Thus the cost of appointing an additional member of staff would be expressed in terms of the cost of the forgone opportunity of instead providing another facility of similar value.

What is the relevance of all this to the provision of nursing services in general and the employment of nursing auxiliaries in particular? Can and should the economic argument be invoked in decision-making relating to the employment nursing auxiliaries?

Although the basic principles of economic analysis have general application, it is necessary to stress that the involvement of nurses at top-level decision-making in health care provision is greater in the UK than in most other countries.

Initially, nursing auxiliaries were employed in this country because of recruitment problems of nurse learners and attrition of learners and qualified nursing staff. A further impetus was provided by the increasing self-consciousness of nursing as a profession. Circumstances have changed recently and there has been a marked reduction in attrition, no doubt due to the general job shortage. There are also more applicants for admission to train in colleges of nursing and midwifery than can be accepted. It can be argued, therefore, that some of the reasons for the employment of nursing auxiliaries have disappeared. None the less, their employment has continued to increase in some areas, whilst it has decreased in others; the recruitment argument has changed to the economic one and I have heard the simple economic argument, 'We can't afford it' advanced to support opposing policies. Some insist that they cannot afford not to employ nursing auxiliaries to supplement the labour force, others state categorically that they cannot afford to employ nursing auxiliaries as their adequate supervision and appropriate deployment are too complex.

There is little doubt that the contribution of this grade of worker is generally well recognised, particularly in the hospital environment. Our current national study of the nursing auxiliary produced findings in support of this statement. Moreover, once established as a recognised work-force, trade union activity would militate against its marked reduction or withdrawal whether this would be deemed desirable or not.

Therefore, it behoves us to invoke the more sophisticated economic analysis I referred to earlier, starting with a careful study of the different types of cost. In the UK, where learners provide a significant proportion of the nursing labour force, comparative average costing of salaries may come out on the side of the learner, as being cheaper than the nursing auxiliary. Extra-duty payments, overtime and other benefits would probably make the nursing auxiliary considerably more expensive at the weekend and on night duty. The marginal cost of providing an extra unit of auxiliary time against an extra unit of qualified time may not be as clear-cut as it appears. Redeployment of qualified staff and its rational allocation based on established needs of patients may be cheaper and more helpful than the overtime deployment of a nursing auxiliary. The opposite may be equally true and each individual situation should be carefully assessed; no general rule will work. Similarly, in estimating the opportunity costs one canot pronounce with any measure of confidence on what one could have gained by not employing an additional nursing auxiliary or, alternatively, by not employing an additional qualified nurse. The individual situation will prompt the right decision but the different costing possibilities should be applied. Professor Spitzer[7] describes the professional as a decision-maker and the auxiliary as an implementer. This may be a useful distinction in rational job allocation which makes economic sense.

There are two root causes of difficulty in making decisions about nurse staffing. First, the many blurred boundaries between the functions of nurses and a wide variety of other people, from the lay public in the form of caring relatives or friends, the domestic, the physiotherapist, the laboratory technician, the doctor and others. The second difficulty, which is related to the first, is the possibility of nurses pricing themselves out of the market, not only by commanding higher salaries, but also by their increasing selectiveness in how they should be employed. Therefore at a time of economic recession there is a temptation to employ the cheapest available pair of hands without regard to benefit or effectiveness.

Cost-benefit and cost-effectiveness are not only relevant but essential concepts in the provision of nursing services. I have already talked about cost and the need to look at all its possible calculations. The economist will certainly give expert assistance in this respect. As far as the calculation of benefit and effectiveness are concerned, the professional must make his or her expert contribution. If the cost side of the economic equation works against the employment of qualified nurses or, for that matter, against the recruitment of learners or the employment of nursing auxiliaries, the professional must provide the balance on the benefit or effectiveness side. Because benefits may have a time lag, they tend to be based on opinions, personal values and assumption rather than factual evidence, thereby losing out on serious consideration. Cost-effectiveness is, therefore, the method of choice in arriving at a decision about level and mix of staff to provide a given nursing service within a given available budget. Professor Cochrane, in his Rock Carling lecture, posited the effectiveness/efficiency dichotomy, which has not yet been fully integrated into economic terminology.[8] It would be more sensible to speak of cost-efficiency rather than cost-effectiveness. A nursing service staffed by fully qualified nurses only may be effective, but we would probably agree that, even if we could afford it, it would not be efficient.

We are left with the most difficult question of all, a question which is as difficult as it is fundamental. It is: what is an efficient nursing service? Attempts to answer the question are not lacking and the nursing literature related to calculation of nursing work-load, nursing establishment, nurse satisfaction and even patient satisfaction is growing rapidly. I do not expect that a definitive answer to that question will ever be found, but I believe that some additional knowledge will be generated by further research, particularly of a type which looks at nursing as part of the wider health care system and which includes in its ambit the recipient of care, as well as his family – the consumer cost referred to earlier. The economic argument must include costs of care which are passed from the public to the private nurse, the costs to the patient and the family. It should also take account of social and emotional costs which are difficult but not impossible to calculate, albeit crudely. This is another professional responsibility with which the economist should expect the professionals to assist him.

A further consideration in the economic argument is the extent of transferability of the worker. Spitzer distinguishes two basic types of auxiliary personnel, those who have certain very specific technical skills, and those who have no such specific skills. Presumably the first type could perform their specific skills repetitively and efficiently, even without supervision. The second type, on the other hand, could undertake a wide variety of tasks. Their deployment could be more flexible but they would require supervision. The economic argument must take these possibilities into account, particularly the cost and feasibility of adequate supervision as well as the cost related to litigation in case of accidents due to inadequate supervision.

This leads to the question of the relationship between professional judgement and economic prudence. I believe that the professional nurse has a responsibility to guard professional standards, not for the sake of professional prestige, but for the sake of patient safety.

Figure 4.1 illustrates some of the choice in staff mix which a manager, operating within a given budget, may have. The example shows a budget of £30,000, and for the sake of simplicity it assumes that one qualified nurse can be obtained for £3,000 per annum and one auxiliary for £1,500 per annum. Thus it can be seen that the manager can, for example, buy eight qualified nurses and four auxiliaries (a), five qualified nurses and ten auxiliaries (b), or two qualified nurses and sixteen auxiliaries (c), as well as many other combinations. If the number of auxiliaries is plotted on the vertical axis, the curve will get steeper as their ratio to qualified nurses increases. I have called the curve the responsibility curve, the reason for which is explained below.

The triangle thus constructed, that is the area bounded by the responsibility curve $R_1 R_2$, must represent the total work to be undertaken by the number and mix of staff shown (Figure 4.2 (a)). Part of this area must be the preserve of qualified nurses, otherwise there would be no need for them. I have called this area the danger zone $O_1 R_2 D$, the point D being the danger point (Figure 4.2 (b)).

to Auxiliaries Within a Given Budget

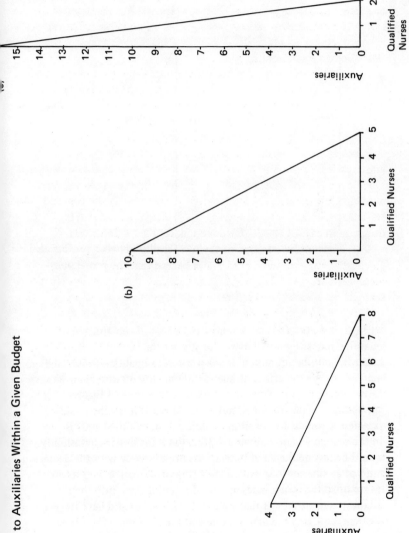

Figure 4.2: Responsibility Curve and Danger Point

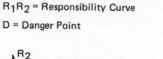

$R_1R_2$ = Responsibility Curve

D = Danger Point

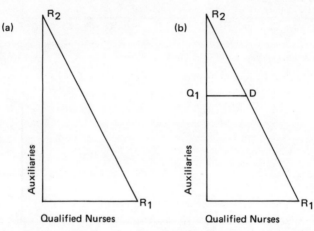

Figures 4.3(a), (b) and (c) show the effect of substitution of qualified nurses by auxiliaries. The steeper the curve that is, the larger the number of auxiliaries in relation to qualified nurses, the more marked will be the effect of one further qualified nurse being absent for whatever reason. Thus, in the extreme example of Figure 4.3(a), the absence of one qualified nurse would result in a substantial transfer of responsibility from qualified to unqualified staff $R_1$ to $R_3$. In the second example, Figure 4.3(b), the transfer of responsibility would be less marked and it decreases progressively with the decreased ratio of auxiliaries to qualified staff (Figure 4.3(c)). Managers are aware of staff absence rates and need to build them into their establishment. I submit that each ward or unit should have its own diagram depicting the danger zone and the staff mix. The diagram would show immediately if the absence of a given number of qualified nurses would result in a responsibility transfer beyond the danger point and, therefore, an encroachment of the unqualified staff into the danger zone. I believe that the size of the danger zone will differ

Figure 4.3: The Effects of Substitution of Qualified Nurses by Auxiliaries

R = Responsibility Curve

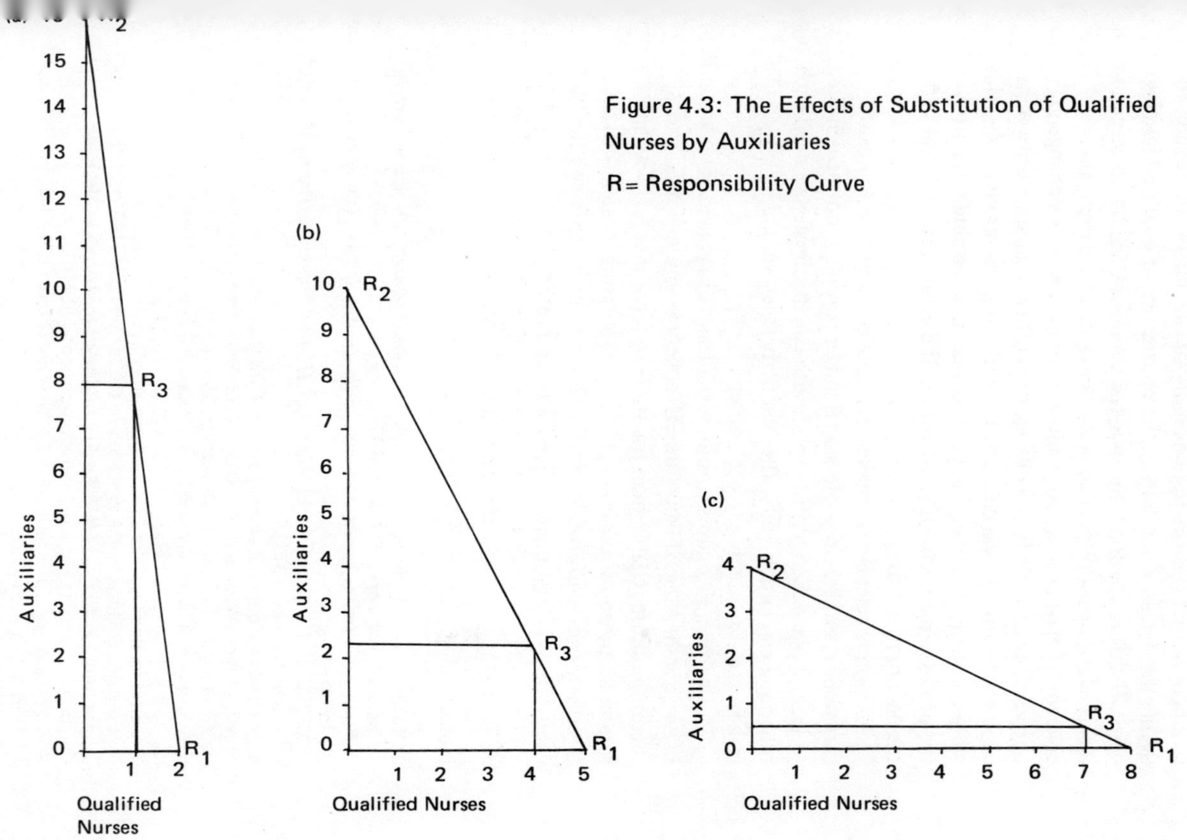

from ward to ward and may even differ over time on the same ward. If the diagram, kept updated, could be displayed at the nursing station and staff absences related to it, it would be an immediate and effective warning signal.

I believe that it is the responsibility of the nursing profession to define the danger zone, that is, the prerogative of qualified nursing work. If this is not done, the demand for nurses will be, in economic terms, elastic with respect to price. As alluded to earlier, the concept of elasticity in economic science relates to the change in one variable as a result of a change in another. If an expensive item can be substituted by a cheaper one without gross disadvantage, this will, of course, be done. The professional must be able to identify the professional result of substitution, the economist will deal with the economic result.

Economic science can make a positive contribution to health care policy, but sound professional judgement must not be demoted to second place. Economists and health care professionals need each other and can enrich each other's activity; they should be supportive rather than threatening to each other.

The economic argument is important and has considerable potential in decision-making. It can work effectively in any direction and is, therefore, more reliable than tradition and sentiment. It warrants serious study and I recommend it as a stimulating challenge to the treasured and comfortable *status quo*. I do not recommend the 'We can't afford it' argument as licence to do nothing.

## Notes

1. Robert Maxwell, *Health Care – The Growing Dilemma,* a McKinsey survey report (New York, McKinsey, 1974).
2. Brian Abel-Smith, *Value for Money in the Health Services* (London, Heinemann, 1976).
3. Michael H. Cooper and J. Culyer (eds.), *Health Economics* (Harmondsworth, Penguin Books, 1973).
4. Michael H. Cooper, *Rationing Health Care* (London, Croom Helm, 1975).
5. A.J. Culyer, *Needs and the National Health Service Economics and Social Choice* (London, Martin Robertson, 1976).
6. C.M. Price, *Welfare Economics in Theory and Practice* (London and Basingstoke, Macmillan, 1977).
7. Walter O. Spitzer, 'The Effect of the Allied Health Professions on Cost Containing Shifts in the Provision of Health Services' (1976). To be published in 1977 in *Priorities for the Use of Resources in Medicine* (Bethesda, USA, Fogarty International Center, 1976).
8. A.L. Cochrane, *Effectiveness and Efficiency* (London, the Nuffield Provincial Hospital Trust, 1973).

# 5 NURSING AUXILIARIES: A PROFESSIONAL PERSPECTIVE IN RELATION TO ROLE AND SUBSEQUENT TRAINING

David Rye

In considering this topic, I have attempted to keep the brief broad in conceptual terms. The professional perspective will be explored in some detail, and will refer to the policy of the Royal College of Nursing regarding nursing auxiliaries employed in the National Health Service. At the same time, I will attempt to analyse and quantify the nursing auxiliary role, with the objective of developing a realistic and meaningful model for training this grade of staff.

For present purposes, the nursing auxiliary role will need to be considered against the background of a multi-specialist involvement in nursing care, i.e. that nurses in this grade are currently operating across a wide range of nursing activity: acute services, psychiatric services, geriatric services, mental handicap, and in the community. Initially, it is important to examine the historical elements, especially in relation to the contribution that nursing auxiliaries have made and are making as an essential part of nursing manpower. In the fields of mental health and mental subnormality, the auxiliary is known as a nursing assistant but the functions are similar.

The definitions for these staff grades in the *Nursing and Midwives Council Handbook* are as follows:

(1) A nursing Auxiliary is a person engaged wholly or mainly on nursing duties (other than in a psychiatric hospital) who has no recognised nursing or midwifery qualification and who is not a student nurse, pupil nurse, or pupil midwife.
(2) A nursing Assistant is a person not being a qualified mental nurse or a Student Mental Nurse or a Pupil Nurse who is engaged in mental nursing duties under the supervision of a qualified mental nurse.

In assessing the contribution that nursing auxiliaries have made over the last 25 years, it is interesting to compare their relative position in numerical terms. In 1949[1] there were 59,529 registered and enrolled nurses and 69,697 learners and auxiliaries. The trained staff comprised 46 per cent of the total while learners and auxiliaries made up the remaining 54 per cent. At that time, learners were 37 per cent of the total and auxiliaries were 17 per cent. These proportions have undergone considerable variability in the intervening years. Learners at one stage represented over 45 per cent of the nursing staff. However, the position in 1975 (latest available statistics) was that there were 131,046 registered and enrolled nurses and 150,454 learners and auxiliaries. The trained staff make up the same percentage of the total that they did in 1949, i.e. 46 per cent. The learners represent only 25 per cent of the total, whilst the remainder of the nursing force is made up of over 100,000 untrained auxiliaries. These are significant statistics, whatever the professional perspective might be. The reality of the situation is that we have a large percentage of the work-force delivering nursing care who are untrained. While on the subject of the balance of staff, it is of interest to note that while registered nurses have risen by 92 per cent, medical consultants have increased by 185 per cent and hospital medical staff by 129 per cent. Almost all consultant appointments have a nursing consequence. Some of the more specialised medical areas have a heavy dependence on trained nursing staff. It can be seen, therefore, that in spite of nurse training advances, it does not seem to have made the impact that was first envisaged. This is particularly so in relation to the training for state enrolment (second-level nurses), which, after all, was introduced as a mechanism for reducing the number of untrained personnel at the bedside. Increasing numbers of people training for the Roll have not offset the number of people being employed as nursing auxiliaries. In essence it is an economic fact that nurses in training are no longer 'cheap labour'. They are now a very expensive commodity and in the last eighteen months this has had impact. Employing authorities seem to be more interested in employing nursing auxiliaries as a means of buying more pairs of hands.

In summing up the historical elements, a final comment: there is no evidence available at the present time on a national basis regarding the effectiveness of the nursing auxiliary. By effectiveness, one may view two dimensions — cost-effectiveness, in terms of manpower planning, and effectiveness in qualitative terms related to the standards of nursing care. I would stress, therefore, the great importance of this particular research project being carried out jointly between the Department of Health and Social Security and the Scottish Home and Health Department. It is a vital piece of work which is long overdue.

## Royal College of Nursing Professional Policy

The RCN has been actively involved over the years in formulating a realistic professional approach to the nursing auxiliary. It does not admit nursing auxiliaries into membership. This subject was debated at this year's Representative Body meeting. The resolution 'that this meeting of the RCN Representative Body requests Council to offer affiliated membership of the RCN to Nursing Auxiliaries' was rejected overwhelmingly. There is no doubt that if the RCN is to retain its credibility as a professional organisation, it cannot receive into membership untrained personnel who are not in training for any of the statutory qualifications. However, the RCN will continue to be involved with and support the Nursing Auxiliaries Association, and the liaison committee which has been formed with them.

Another debated professional issue was associated with the number of the nursing auxiliaries in the NHS, and especially the balance of staff in ward and departmental nursing teams. The policy which emerged as a result of a debate on the phasing out of auxiliaries was that numbers should be reduced to a level allowing a balanced nursing team. What is balance? It clearly would be unrealistic in the short term to talk about abolishing this grade altogether. It is worth pointing out that at a time of high unemployment, when it is becoming very difficult for trained nurses to obtain jobs, this becomes a highly contentious issue, professionally, politically and economically. Clearly it points to the lack of strategic manpower planning in the NHS as far as nursing services are concerned. There is increasing concern from the RCN membership on this issue. They feel strongly about the number of nurses being trained who find themselves without jobs after qualifying. They believe that the revenue costs would not be greatly increased if state enrolled nurses were employed instead of nursing auxiliaries.

I refer to the Royal College of Nursing's evidence to the Committee on Nursing[2]  (The Briggs Committee[3]):

67. The spectrum of activities encompassed by the generic term 'nursing' is so wide that it provides opportunity for those with a variety of aptitudes, abilities, skills and inclinations. At one end of the spectrum it represents an instinctive response to human need which is demonstrated by those who have, and require, no training; the mother who cares for her infant child, and who also cares for

members of her family through minor ailments. At the other end it demands specialist knowledge and skills and the ability to exercise judgements at a high level; this presupposes studies in basic sciences, in the behavioural sciences as well as in clinical subjects and the acquisition of a wide range of technical skills (p.17, para. 67).

93. Nursing Aides (who would take the place of the present Nursing Auxiliaries and Nursing Assistants) should be accepted from the age of 17 years and must be given an approved course of preparation. The 'School' would be responsible for the organisation of this period of preparation which should include a planned induction to the institution in which the Aide is to work.

94. A suitable preparation as an introduction to nursing might be based on the course for the nursing certificate of the St John Ambulance Association, St Andrew's Ambulance Association and the British Red Cross Society. This of course would be organised by the 'School'. Those entrants who had already obtained the joint organisations' certificate within the previous two years, would be exempted from this part of the course.

95. Subsequently the Nursing Aide would receive in-service training for the first six months of employment, possibly amounting to half-a-day each fortnight.

96. Nursing Aides would work under the direction and supervision of trained nurses: they would be the nurses' helpers (p.24, paras. 93-6).

207. The RCN plan emphasises that all who contribute to nursing care should receive preparation for their work. Opportunity should be made available for all those who had received no formal preparation to take the course of preparation for the nursing certificate suggested as appropriate for the 'nursing aide' in paragraph 94. Discussions should be initiated without delay with the three organisations to determine the help which they could give in this matter. Additionally, all employing authorities should be required, within a given period of time, to offer in-service training to these members of staff (p.52, para. 207(i), Nursing Auxiliaries and Assistants).

With reference to quantitative analysis, the number of nursing auxiliaries is inextricably linked with the way student nurse training is funded at present. The most recent work on nursing auxiliaries in terms of their role is to be found in the *Report* of the Committee on Nursing (Briggs) which highlights the variation in the role and training of these workers. It produced some useful statistical information as well as making recommendations related to the training of nursing aides. The *Report* proposed that these nursing aides would succeed the present nursing auxiliaries and assistants, if and when the recommendations were implemented. It is worth considering these recommendations again presently because it appears that Briggs legislation is now imminent, with the setting up of the co-ordinating committee and working groups that will investigate detail and make proposals on which further legislation will be based. Again we are back to the economic perspective in decision-making terms, and it seems likely that decisions about aides will hinge on whether or not nurses in training are counted as part of the funded nursing establishment.

In its evidence to Briggs, the RCN stated that

> it is firmly of the opinion that training for a professional qualification must be separated from service and that an essential factor in achieving this is by the provision of student grants instead of a salary disguised as a 'training allowance' from an employing authority.

The Briggs Committee itself suggested that this could be achieved by a cross-accounting system. Students could be financed through an educational authority, but account would have to be taken of their manpower contribution during the training period. This is a very different perspective to having a student who is supernumary to manpower requirements. However, whatever model is adopted, it seems probable that there will be a continuous increase in the number of nursing auxiliaries.

## An Analysis of the Role

I introduce here some detailed information on work that I was involved with as a Director of Nurse Education, and give some specific examples of role analysis in relation to specialty areas of nursing care. I think it appropriate to include examples from the general field of hospital nursing, but also to make reference to the Community Nursing Service. It should also be pointed out that there could be a particular role for the nursing auxiliary in mental handicap facilities.

In analysing the role of the nursing auxiliary, I include in this paper working examples of job descriptions produced after considerable discussion and negotiation between the School of Nursing and service personnel. They contain interesting material in the context of attempted decision-making about the clinical involvement of the nursing auxiliary. This reflects on how far an organisation must go in developing the role, and then the subsequent training which is necessary. There must be a cut-off point. Many trained staff, especially enrolled nurses, are sensitive about technical nursing care carried out by nursing auxiliaries that impinges on the trained nurse's role. The job description following, of the general division in particular, attempts to divide the nursing care into three categories:

Section A being a category which could be described as basic nursing care skills which have to be taught before undertaking these tasks in relation to patient care.

Section B highlights the need for a degree of flexibility in the clinical situation by defining those procedures that could be carried out at the discretion of the Ward Sister or Charge Nurse in consultation with the Nursing Officer.

Section C categorises those procedures which under no circumstances must be undertaken by the nursing auxiliary.

The job description is used as a tool in developing operational policies in relation to role. Critics may argue that this type of analysis is too task-orientated and that the definition of 'role' should be more patient-centred. This is a controversial issue which may provoke much discussion.

## The Development of the Model for Training the Nursing Auxiliary

*Example: General Division*

SECTION A

Nursing auxiliaries must have received instruction before undertaking the following:

(1)   (a)   Reception – orientation to ward.
      (b)   Assist with admission procedures/discharge/transfer to and from hospital and other departments in conjunction with trained staff. Appropriate duties to include care and listing of

clothing and property, particularly dentures and spectacles.

(2) (a) General bed-making (making occupied beds and cots; stripping and making unoccupied beds and cots; admission bed; bed for patient sitting upright, bed for patient lying flat or recumbent).

(b) Lifting, turning and moving patient.

(c) Use and care of bedding, bed linen, bed accessories, cradles, ambulift, etc.

(3) (a) Bed bathing; general bathing; washing of hair; care of mouth, dentures, skin, nails, hands, feet; general hygiene.

(b) Shaving patients (toilet only, not pre-operative).

(c) Care of pressure areas – prevention of bedsores.

(d) Assist learners or trained staff with the care of incontinent patients.

(e) Assist learners or trained staff with the care of helpless patients.

(f) Changing infant napkins.

(4) (a) Giving of bedpans and urinals.

(b) Obtaining specimens (i.e. sputum, faeces and 24-hourly urine), labelling, and taking them to the laboratory where necessary.

(c) Recording of Fluid Intake and Urine Output Charts under supervision.

(5) (a) Preparation of patients for meals in all age groups.

(b) Assist with service of meals – feeding helpless patients.

(c) Serving drinks and beverages at discretion of ward sister.

(d) Care of mouth of conscious patients only.

(6) (a) Care of ambulant patients – escorting patients to other wards and departments, dressing and undressing patients and getting them in and out of bed.

(b) Assist patients to bathroom, WC, commode and sanichairs.

(c) Weighing patients, reporting to trained staff and keeping records.

(d) Chaperoning patients in clinics.

(7) Care of infectious patients and treatment of infectious property, equipment, etc. if accompanied by learner and/or trained staff.

(8) (a) Simple bandaging.

(b) Assist trained member of staff with preparing patients for operation.

(9) Answering telephone; taking, recording and transmitting messages.

(10) (a) Clean and prepare nursing equipment (in non-training hospitals only).
    (b) Care of all hospital equipment and furniture.
    (c) Clean and tidy clinical equipment and storage cupboards, excluding cupboards for dangerous drugs and scheduled poisons.
    (d) Tidying contents of patients' lockers.

(11) Assist with last offices under supervision.

(12) Assist in the keeping of specified records and charts, e.g. weight and fluid charts.

(13) (a) Assist with occupational and diversional therapy, including recreation, sport and play.
    (b) Assist with rehabilitative measures, e.g. crutches, walking frames.
    (c) Assist with exercises.

(14) First aid: action in case of cardiac arrest; action in case of fire in ward/department.

## SECTION B

The following procedures must only be carried out: (a) at the discretion of the sister in charge, in consultation with the Nursing Officer of the unit concerned; (b) if the nursing auxiliary is asked to do so by the nurse in charge of the ward, and *full instructions by trained staff* have been given on the duty in question; (c) provided student and pupil nurses in the ward are given opportunity to gain the necessary experience.

(1) Taking temperature, pulse and respiration.

(2) Testing of urine.

(3) Local application of creams and ointment.

(4) Changing of colostomy bags.

(5) Giving inhalations.
    N.B.  Staff working in a specialised department, e.g. theatre, out-patients, ICU and maternity, may be requested to carry out more advanced procedure.

## SECTION C

Nursing auxiliaries are *not allowed* to undertake the following:

(1) Checking and giving drugs.

(2) Dressings.

(3) Give injections: hypodermic; intramuscular.

(4) Assist with or change intravenous infusions.

(5)  Gastric tube-feeding and aspiration of naso-gastric tube.
(6)  Catheterisation or changing of bladder drainage bags.
(7)  Observation or care of the unconscious patient.
(8)  Preparation of infant feeds.
(9)  Use of oxygen — changing of cylinders, observation of amount used and rate of flow, use of tents, etc.
(10)  Giving medical information to patients or relatives.
(11)  Application of traction.
(12)  Recording blood pressure.
(13)  Giving of enemas or suppositories.
      N.B.  Sisters will be held personally responsible for unauthorised duties undertaken by nursing auxiliaries in their ward or department.

*Example: Community Division*

NURSING AUXILIARIES

Report to Community Nursing Officer.
Responsible to Community Nursing Sister.

*Work-load authorised and delegated by District Nursing Sister*

Nursing auxiliaries must have received instruction before undertaking the following:
(1)  Observation of the patient and his/her total needs, including stress situations in the family, so that these can be referred to the District Nursing Sister.
(2)  Bathing patients in their own homes: (i) in the bathroom (ii) in bed.
(3)  Washing patient's hair.
(4)  Care of mouth, dentures, skin, nails, hands and feet, general hygiene.
(5)  Care of pressures areas — prevention of bedsores.
(6)  Dressing and undressing patients and getting them in and out of bed.
(7)  Lifting, turning and moving patients.
(8)  Care of ambulant incontinent patients.
(9)  Assist trained staff with the care of incontinent patients.
(10)  Assist trained staff with the care of helpless patients.
(11)  Assist with rehabilitation of patients, e.g. use of walking frames, walking sticks and crutches. Passive exercises.
(12)  Assist patients to bathroom, toilet and commode.
(13)  Simple dressing.
(14)  Simple bandaging.
(15)  Reporting on patient's condition to District Nursing Sister.

(16)　The taking of patient's temperature in certain conditions so that relevant information can be given to the District Nursing Sister when there is doubt about a patient's progress.

(17)　Ensuring the safety of the patient's environment.

(18)　To make available to the patient those items that are necessary for his/her total comfort, e.g. drinks in readily accessible place together with reading glasses, and a bell to attract attention of the family, and the means of diversional therapy, e.g. papers, books, etc.

In discussing role analysis, it seems useful to concentrate on detailed information, using job descriptions which have been utilised and tested, and which have been modified after evaluation. When one attempts to answer the question 'What should a nursing auxiliary be doing in practical terms?' certain conflicts arise. One of the most difficult areas is associated with the variable training overlap of the nursing auxiliary and the trained nurse, whether registered or enrolled. Indeed, one of the barriers to developing models of training for the nursing auxiliary has been the somewhat over-cautious and protective attitude of trained staff. Comments are made like, 'Is a third tier of training really necessary?'

Some problems are not open to immediate resolution, and there must be a flexible approach at local level in order to identify and resolve them. If one compares the difference in role for the auxiliary between specialties such as acute services, mental handicap and community, there is quite clearly a common core content which can be isolated, hence a common introductory programme for mixed groups of nursing auxiliaries is viable. The establishment of nursing auxiliary training very often hinges on release of staff from their hours of duty; how cost-effective is this? The training model which is adopted is all-important. It also becomes very important to have a consensus view throughout a health district on how far the training should be taken, and in identifying those procedures which must fall outside the remit of the nursing auxiliary. Historically, this has always been a very difficult situation to control. There has been a lack of clearly defined operational policies on the part of employing authorities. I believe that it is possible to both to standardise and to develop a meaningful interpretation of the nursing auxiliary role and subsequently the training required, provided that there is the will. It involves many people in detailed work which necessitates forward planning and impinges on the nurse educator, nurse manager and nurse practitioner. Each must be committed to the basic philosophy that all personnel adopting a caring role should be trained accordingly.

The training model itself must be adopted as soon as there has been adequate role definition and a consensus view reached. The major problems involved in developing in-service training programmes for nursing auxiliary staff have been associated with two or three major areas. One of these is the criteria used for selection of candidates. Is there a minimum standard acceptable? If so, what criteria are used in assessing the individual's potential for carrying out specific clinical tasks which involve manual and interactional skills? What sort of testing would be useful? Intelligence testing, personality testing, the testing of motivation? These issues, already well defined and documented, remain unsolved.

Another major problem is linking the training with the immediate commencement of the nursing auxiliary's employment. The two should be coterminous, and in practical terms this is often difficult to achieve. In 1962, Beck stated:

> If untrained auxiliary nurses are employed, it is essential that they receive planned and not haphazard on-the-job training. This must be simple and straightforward — possibly similar to forms of training within industry — but it must be emphasised that the auxiliary nurse is dealing with human beings, and this aspect of her work must be constantly kept before her. There is a certain danger that on-the-job training may tend to stress equipment and activities, rather than people. This must be avoided.[4]

It does seem remarkable that although none of this is new, the development of auxiliary training is still, relatively speaking, retarded. We have not had the growth in relation to carrying out work on the role and subsequent training programmes, though we have had continuous growth in numbers. In manpower terms it is bound to be affected by any new legislation that emerges in relation to nurse training. It is therefore appropriate to give more attention to this subject, if for no other reason than to enhance the standards of care.

### Conclusion

I have attempted to outline the professional perspective with special reference to the Royal College of Nursing policy. At the same time I have tried to point out other important issues associated with analysing the role of the nursing auxiliary. Essentially, I have put forward a practical approach to this complex subject rather than a hypothetical one. In my view, nursing auxiliary employment and training is a practical problem. There is scope for the employing authorities to develop meaningful training models, provided that there is the drive and motivation to do so on the part of senior nursing staff. It is their responsibility to formulate and implement operational policies of this type.

Much of what I have proposed is based on my own experience, and is in no way necessarily unique or original. At least it is an example of an approach that has been made in a large health care district to come to grips with meeting the needs of untrained nursing personnel. Frances Beck's words seem as appropriate now as they were in 1962:

> This paper has reviewed some points and problems associated with functions, training and utilisation of auxiliary nursing personnel. While no easy solutions are available, an attempt has been made to indicate the kinds of considerations that must be taken into account in individual circumstances if any new approach is to be made towards solving any of the problems facing us in this field.[5]

It can perhaps be said, in conclusion, that any new approach is likely to be the result of careful analysis, with consideration of many and varied factors. It is likely that each nursing situation (whether considered nationally, by institution or by agency) will require its special solution, because the factors specific to each situation will vary. No solution will be found without consideration of the work of all personnel contributing to the task which must be studied in relation to medicine and its foreseeable development.

## Notes

1. Royal College of Nursing, 'The Effect of Financial Cutbacks in the National Health Service on the Standards of Care' (London, January 1977).
2. Royal College of Nursing, *Evidence to the Committee on Nursing* (Briggs) (1971).
3. Department of Health and Social Security and Scottish Home and Health Department, *Report of the Committee on Nursing* (Chairman: Asa Briggs), Cmnd 5115 (London, HMSO, 1972).
4. Frances S. Beck, 'Finding a new approach in the Training and Use of Auxiliary Nursing Personnel', World Health Organisation, paper, Spain, 1962.
5. Beck, op.cit.

# 6 NURSING AUXILIARIES – TRAINING FOR WHAT? THE DILEMMA OF NURSING EDUCATORS

Thomas Snee

## Introduction

The definitions for a nursing auxiliary and a nursing assistant as laid down in the Nurses and Midwives Whitley Council Handbook are:

(a) a nursing auxiliary is a person who has no recognised nursing or midwifery qualification and who is not a student nurse, pupil midwife or pupil nurse, who is engaged wholly or mainly on nursing duties in a hospital (other than in a psychiatric hospital) under the supervision of a qualified nurse or midwife;

(b) a nursing assistant is a person not being a qualified mental nurse or a student mental nurse or a pupil nurse who is engaged in mental nursing duties in a hospital under the supervision of a qualified mental nurse.[1]

In 1977 the grade of nursing auxiliary was officially introduced into the community nursing services.[2] Prior to this date a variety of grades of ancillary nursing staff were working as a back-up service to qualified nurses in the community.

In the *Report of the Committee on Nursing* (the Briggs Report)[3] it was stated in paragraph 85b that this group of people referred to as nursing aides had no professional training. Patients may call them nurse and they enable service to the patient to be maintained and improved, not least at night, but they are outside the profession. Briggs went on to say that his committee believed that the education of nursing aides was a matter of considerable urgency and recommended the institution of a planned scheme of in-service training (paragraphs 336-41).

Any member of staff, of whatever grade, working in the Health Service, who is responsible (no matter how little) for the delivery of care and who is an integral member of the health care team, must be prepared for the jobs he or she actually does. That preparation is something which can be debated at length and, in relation to nursing auxiliaries, it might be more pertinent to consider not so much what they can or should do, but what they cannot or should not do.

## History and Growth Rate

In the early 1950s there was an apparent need to provide some form of supporting service to the trained nursing staff. In view of this the basic grade of nursing auxiliary was first commended to the National Health Service in 1955.

After an initial slow start the number of nursing auxiliaries and assistants has grown considerably. Table 6.1 gives a comparison over a ten-year period, for England only.

Table 6.1: Nursing Auxiliaries and Assistants Growth Rate (in whole-time equivalents)

|  | 1965 | 1971 | 1972 | 1973 | 1974 | 1975 |
|---|---|---|---|---|---|---|
| Hospital | 45,990 | 54,559 | 60,865 | 62,590 | 66,734 | 77,003 |
| Community | 212 | 1,184 | 1,485 | 1,656 | 2,391 | 2,391 |

Source: DHSS *Health and Personal Social Services Statistics for England*.

Similarly, from Table 6.2 comparative growth figures of auxiliaries in hospital *vis-à-vis* the trained nursing staff and student and pupil nurses can be seen.

Table 6.2: Comparative Growth Rate – Hospital (whole-time equivalents)

| Total | 1965 | 1971 | 1972 | 1973 | 1974 | 1975 |
|---|---|---|---|---|---|---|
| Registered nurses | 65,711 | 74,520 | 76,956 | 76,057 | 76,856 | 83,329 |
| Enrolled nurses | 20,366 | 35,898 | 38,674 | 39,327 | 40,354 | 44,480 |
| Student and pupil nurses | 64,215 | 67,659 | 71,875 | 73,805 | 72,826 | 75,889 |
| Other nursing staff | 45,990 | 54,559 | 60,865 | 62,590 | 66,734 | 77,003 |

Source: DHSS, *Health and Personal Social Services Statistics for England*.

## Role

The auxiliary fulfils a multiplicity of roles, the preparation for which is questionable. From the limited written evidence available there are two specific areas which can be used to illustrate this point.

(1) Abstract of Efficiency Studies in the Hospital Service No.136 describes a study on relieving nurses of non-nursing duties which was carried out in 1970. One particular aspect of the study was to monitor the number of visits by nursing staff to the X-ray department. Over a four-hour period 31 visits were made, averaging one every 8 minutes, and 25 per cent of these visits were carried out by nursing auxiliaries. As a result of the study a decision was made to extend the portering services, thereby relieving nursing auxiliaries of some of their messenger duties and releasing them for patient care.

(2) In a survey carried out by the North East Metropolitan Regional Hospital Board in March 1974 on supporting services and non-nursing duties undertaken by nurses at one maternity hospital, the fact was highlighted that nursing auxiliaries were employed to provide the night staff with a meal service and others to clean toilets, baths and showers. By the purchase of a vending machine and microwave oven on one hand and the transfer of the cleaning duties to the domestic services on the other, time available for direct patient care was increased.

The variation in the studies of auxiliaries indicates that health authorities are interpreting the role to fit their own perceived needs and this can work to the advantage of the health service. *Hospital Abstract* No.117 (1968) described the allocation of duties between trained nursing staff, auxiliary nurses and domestic staff at a large general hospital. The salient part of this study was in highlighting the correct deployment of staff, particularly illustrated by the fact that much of the work at that time carried out by qualified nurses in the out-patient department could be carried out by nursing auxiliaries or clerical staff. On completion of the study it was possible, by changing the hours of the domestic staff and reallocating the duties of auxiliaries and clerical staff, to transfer one charge nurse, two full-time staff nurses and one part-time staff nurse to the wards and to employ four nursing auxiliaries in their place.

Possibly one of the factors influencing the apparently indiscriminate appointment of nursing auxiliaries has been the lack of guidance available for the training of the nursing auxiliary, although one cannot dismiss the fact that there is expediency in appointing unqualified nursing personnel who can be absorbed into the nursing team very quickly.

## The Difficulties

(1) Date of commencement. Because of the need to fill jobs it is not easy to arrange a common date of entry for nusing auxiliaries, although it is encouraging to note that some employers are insisting on just this. With the recruitment of auxiliaries on an individual basis some health authorities might question the need to allocate the resources needed for an orientation period, but hopefully an acceptable compromise can be reached.

(2) Adaptability. Many auxiliaries are housewives with home commitments and no previous experience of nursing or possibly any other kind of paid work, but they are mature and responsible people used to caring for others. The support and counselling needed initially may be considerable.

(3) Supporting nursing staff. In some parts of the country there is a dearth of qualified nursing staff and it is in these areas that the auxiliaries may well be exposed to responsibility for which they are unprepared.

(4) Teaching personnel. Some health authorities have appointed teaching staff with a specific remit for nursing auxiliary training but these are in a minority. Where there is no specifically appointed teacher to this particular role the teaching must be done on a somewhat *ad hoc* basis.

(5) Service versus education. The service managers have a responsibility to provide an adequate standard of patient care and the dichotomy between providing this care and ensuring by means of training that the care is effective can be a very real concern to them. This is particularly pertinent in the case of nursing auxiliaries. With the ever-increasing demands on qualified nurses it becomes more difficult to release nursing auxiliaries for training purposes. This can, to a degree, include on-the-job training.

(6) Flexibility of approach. Because of the trend to recruit for an individual job, the employer does not always see the need to devise a job description which allocates specific duties to the auxiliary.

## How can These Difficulties Be Overcome?

### Guidance

In 1955 a guidance paper which dealt with courses of instruction for nursing assistants in psychiatric and mental subnormality hospitals in England and Wales was published by the then Ministry of Health.[4]

The recommendations within that document were sufficiently flexible to allow for wide discretion in the detailed planning of courses of instruction. It was indicated, however, that if national certificates were to be awarded the course should have a degree of validity which would be recognised throughout the country and that if this were to be so, it was essential that the courses should obtain a reasonable minimum standard. It is significant that in many psychiatric and subnormality hospitals this guidance document is still in use. In 1962 the Scottish Home and Health Department issued a memorandum on the duties and training of nursing auxiliaries,[5] which was subsequently updated in 1970.[6] The document considered that training for nursing auxiliaries was essential, and that training should be organised on a hospital or group basis and be given as soon as practicable after the nursing auxiliary had taken up employment. Introductory training courses should be of about one week's duration followed by a period of in-service training. It is also suggested that one member of the senior administrative nursing staff should be responsible for organising and co-ordinating the instruction and on-the-job training.

Apart from these documents, little guidance emerged from any official source which might help authorities in the preparation of the nursing auxiliary for his or her role.

There was publication of a further guidance circular from the Scottish Home and Health Department earlier this year[7] and a circular giving comprehensive advice on auxiliary training is in preparation by the Department of Health and Social Security. It is hoped that this will be available to the service in England at an early date after consultation.

*Recruitment and Training*

Nursing auxiliaries are normally recruited for a specific job and invariably this recruitment is made from the local vicinity. Because of home ties it is often found that auxiliaries tend to stay in post for many years. This in itself can give a degree of stability to a job, but because of familiarity can at times also create a feeling on both the auxiliary and trained nurse's part that there is a greater importance attached to the job than was originally meant.

This can only be perpetuated because of the undefined parameters of the auxiliaries' responsibilities.

The present position is that in the United Kingdom, recruitment and training of nursing auxiliaries varies according to local policies. Many health authorities have introduced schemes of training which are highly commendable and designed to equip the auxiliary for the role she is to fill, whereas others provide only an introduction to the work and working environment. Nigel Malin[8] illustrated this aspect and drew attention to the feelings of vulnerability nursing auxiliaries felt when exposed to patients, particularly in the mental subnormality fields, without adequate preparation. The fact that auxiliaries tend to be recruited as and when the need arises can work against effective training schemes. As previously stated, it is unlikely that health authorities can afford to deploy one senior member of nursing staff to mount an orientation period of training for one nursing auxiliary at a time. Also there is the problem of those auxiliaries who only work a few nights or occasional evenings during the week. Barrow-clough and Pinel[9] identified this problem very lucidly and attempted to draw some guidelines on how to organise a programme of instruction with a degree of flexibility to meet all needs. Similarly Jean Snape, describing the night nursing service in Liverpool,[10] highlighted the problem of induction and follow-up training of nursing auxiliaries engaged solely for that night service. The auxiliaries appointed were allocated to day duty for a period of orientation and training before being attached to a district nurse on night duty for supervised instruction. Eventually the nursing auxiliary was allocated a patient with whom she remained for up to 4 weeks. By preparing auxiliaries in this manner it ensured that they had a far more meaningful part to play in the delivery of care than would have been realised otherwise.

Since reorganisation of the NHS in 1974 and publication of the revised structure in nurse education departments,[11] the training needs of auxiliaries have become the responsibility of the Director of Nurse Education. This in itself has caused concern in the nursing profession, concern based on the fact that by firmly placing the instruction of auxiliaries within the school of nursing it could be interpreted that a third grade of qualified nurse would emerge. This is simply not the case, but what does emerge is the need for clear and unequivocal official guidance on the preparation of nursing auxiliaries for their role. This guidance will not stand on its own but needs complementing by the clear policies determined by the individual employing authorities.

*Principles of Training.* The philosophy on training as seen by the Department of Health and Social Security is that auxiliaries should be prepared for the specific jobs for which they have been recruited.

This means that a generic training scheme for all auxiliaries is unnecessary. The guidance document being prepared by the department should not be interpreted as a formal syllabus of training. The need for training and identification of the elements within that training will be within the agreed policy of individual health authorities and will vary according to local circumstances.

*Common Core of Training.* Although there will be no need for a generic training scheme, there will be a common core of instruction needed by all nursing auxiliaries and it is hoped when courses of instruction are being organised it may be possible for auxiliaries through the various fields of nursing care to study together for this part. The common core will embrace subjects like confidentiality of patients' records, this particular aspect being very pertinent when one considers that many auxiliaries will be recruited from the local environment and may know the patients for whom they are caring. Other subjects which might be included in the common core are the communications networks, both written (patient records are part of the written communication network) and verbal, fire precautions and action in case of fire, procedures related to accidents to patients, relatives and staff, and being conversant with complaints procedures.

*Specific Study.* In addition to the common core of instruction auxiliaries should embark on a series of specific study periods orientated to the work in which they are engaged. These ongoing periods should be orientated to giving the auxiliary sufficient insight into the specialty so that their role as a helper to the qualified nurse becomes more meaningful.

*Record of Instruction.* In the helper role the auxiliary will be responsible for carrying out certain routine practical procedures, and it is suggested that employing authorities devise a record of instruction to suit their individual needs and that the supervisor and auxiliary should sign the record when both feel proficiency in a certain procedure has been achieved. This record would remain in the possession of the auxiliary and serve as a basis of instruction if movement to different departments is anticipated. If the auxiliary moves to another employing authority, the new authority would need to satisfy itself that the auxiliary was proficient in previously learned procedures after local practices had been explained and before new procedures were taught. In giving an indication of the procedures which might be considered for inclusion in the work of the nursing auxiliary, it is appreciated that some senior nurses may wish to add other items and this will depend on local policy. Any decision made, however, will have to be in the light of other resources, such as the grades of supporting staff available and a clear definitive picture of the role into which it is envisaged that the auxiliary will fit.

## Degree of Responsibility

No matter what decisions are made on the training for the auxiliaries' role, they must be fully conversant with a maximum and minimum level of responsibility expected. Parameters must be clearly defined by the employing authority. One way of achieving this would be by designing a job description which would set out those tasks which the auxiliary is permitted to carry out.

The objectives indicated in this chapter can only be achieved by the total commitment of those responsible for both education and service needs and, unless the guidance lines are agreed, confusion about auxiliaries' roles will continue to exist. The role of the auxiliary can to a degree be somewhat controversial and Helen Sparrow highlighted this in an article which gave a personal interpretation of how the auxiliary might fulfil her role in the community nursing services.[12] She outlined a range of duties which the auxiliary might perform and these ranged from the giving of specific injections to the dressing of leg ulcers. Although it was clearly stated that courses of in-service training were held at regular periods and followed up by half-study days, also that record books were kept showing the auxiliary's progress and lectures attended, the article triggered off in subsequent correspondence a considerable degree of argument and controversy.[13]

Nurse educationalists have not always been involved in the preparation of nursing auxiliaries and even now only a small proportion are actively engaged in their training. Despite the guidance that has been issued apportioning the responsibility for nursing auxiliary training, there are still many parts of the country where lines are somewhat blurred when it comes to taking an initiative in setting up a course of instruction or training because the recommended arrangements in the reorganisation circular[14] have not been implemented.

## Future Directions

Where are we going? The present economic climate is forcing all employers, the National Health Service among them, to look critically at their manpower resources and the manner in which they are deployed. It is possible that the future could bring a different mix of qualified staff and auxiliaries, but the present numbers and proportion to total of the latter are such that it is essential that we should fully and properly use them. This means that they must be utilised to their full capacity, be given adequate instruction and have adequate support and counselling from the qualified staff to whom they are accountable and also to be recognised as a member of the team. The contribution made to patient care by nursing auxiliaries is not always recognised, but quite often it is the auxiliary who has the closest contact with the patient. The nursing profession is probably in a better position now than ever before to ensure that this contribution is fostered to a degree whereby the auxiliary, through definition of role and training for it, integrates more readily with the team and is provided with greater job satisfaction. When this is achieved the auxiliary will no longer remain a dilemma for education.

## Notes

1. Whitley Councils for the Health Services, *Nurses and Midwives Handbook.*
2. Department of Health and Social Security, Advance Letter (NM) 2/77.
3. Department of Health and Social Security and Scottish Home and Health Department, *Report of the Committee on Nursing,* Cmnd 5115 (London, HMSO, 1972).
4. HM (55) 49.
5. SHM 62/78.
6. SHM 70/1970.
7. NHS Circular No. 1977 (Gen) 35.
8. *Nursing Mirror,* Vol. 143, No. 14.
9. *Nursing Mirror,* 17 July 1975.
10. Practice Team 1973 (284-6).
11. HRC 74/11.
12. *Queen's Nursing Journal* (July 1976).
13. *Queen's Nursing Journal* (November 1976).
14. HRC 74/11.

# 7 AUXILIARIES AS RE-ABLISTS: A MULTI-DISCIPLINARY DIMENSION

Margaret Hawker and Monnica Stewart

Therapists are acutely aware of the growing opinion that it is their
duty to divide the work of providing therapeutic services and to
share responsibility with new kinds of workers in their fields.
These pressures are not entirely welcome for they call upon
therapists to change familiar and generally satisfying styles of
practice, to relinquish tasks regarded as important and to
assume new responsibilities for co-ordinating their efforts with
those of a still unfamiliar category of worker. This uneasiness
is augmented by the fact that many important questions about
the process of sharing remain largely unanswered. There is still
little real consensus among professional therapists about the
appropriate answers to such practical questions as: 'Who should
do what — how will the professional and assistant be different?'
It would be comfortable to postpone change until these questions
have been thoroughly answered, but the urgency of the demand
for new patterns of practice is inescapable.[1]

This quotation from an article by Dr Nancy Watts, a physical
therapist and director of educational studies in Boston, USA, was
written six years ago but has very real relevance for the dilemma
facing the remedial therapy professions in the United Kingdom today.
Remedial helpers are providing a growing proportion of our
work-force and our problems regarding their deployment have much
similarity with those of the nursing profession in the employment
of nursing auxiliaries. The list of topics submitted by delegates for
discussion at the workshop makes this abundantly clear.

We are being forced to look at such factors as job descriptions,
overlapping responsibilities, interdependency, supervision, ratios
of qualified to unqualified staff and that vexed question of training.
It is crucial that our professions reach a decision on criteria for
training and understand that if assistants are not given special
knowledge and education, they weaken the standard of the
professions as a whole.

The British Association of Occupational Therapists has taken the

initiative and set up a national training for its own professional
helpers. However, a common core training programme prepared by a
Joint Working Party of the three professions of physiotherapy,
occupational therapy and remedial gymnastics has met with a good
deal of reaction, particularly from physiotherapists.

## How Will the Assistant and Professional Be Different?

There is still a great deal of ambivalence concerning the deployment
of helpers. To a number of us, particularly in the physiotherapy
profession, 'aides or helpers' are an emotive subject and their
employment is regarded as a threat, leading to eventual dilution of
the service. Others quite genuinely see them as a means of separating
the qualified therapist from direct contact with the patient which
for so many therapists provides the greatest personal satisfaction
and reward.

There has been little consensus agreement on the assistant's role
and function and for the most part her work tends to be fairly tightly
circumscribed within the boundaries of each profession, and although
there is some overlapping there is little general enthusiasm for the
concept of a multi-disciplinary worker. It is still possible to obtain
from the Chartered Society of Physiotherapy a leaflet entitled
'Duties In A Physiotherapy Department That May be Delegated To
Personnel Other Than Physiotherapists', and in many such
departments, the aide or helper is regarded as someone who
carries out humdrum tasks of a standard routine nature, dealing with
such material things as counting linen or cleaning apparatus. In these
situations there is little opportunity for helpers to build up
relationships with individual patients, to make decisions or to use
initiative. Alternatively, in times of acute shortage, helpers have
been used as partly trained therapists taking over certain treatment
procedures. This not only places unfair responsibility on supportive
personnel, but lays the trained therapist open to the very situation
she most wants to avoid, that in times of economic stringency,
employing authorities will recruit semi-skilled assistants in place
of qualified staff.

## The Introduction of 'Re-ablists' to a Department of Geriatric Medicine

It is at this point that it is appropriate to introduce the subject of
're-ablists'; to describe a project which was initiated in 1964 and
which has developed over the years as an integral part of the pattern

of support of patients in the Department of Geriatric Medicine at Edgware General Hospital; and finally to discuss some of the implications of this experiment, in what might well be called community participation. For the professional members of the department's team, the experience has been both rewarding and salutary, for it has forced us to look afresh at established practices and traditional lines of thought through eyes that have not grown dim with custom.

The objectives of any department of geriatric medicine are to try and enable its elderly patients to find a sense of volition and purpose, to regain lost physical capabilities and to find again a sense of worth and some level of emotional competence.

To achieve this requires a more personally orientated service than is essential for patients whose hospital stay is relatively brief. Necessary too is a therapeutic environment where the emphasis is on *support* rather than *care*: for support implies expectation of initiative and effort and the possibility of achievement, whereas care tends to be seen in terms of custody and dependence. In such an environment effort can be directed towards preserving individual life-styles and organising activities that provide stimulus, give opportunities for choice and decision-making and foster social relationships. At the same time, practise in simple self-help activities can be encouraged, so that each patient is able to achieve his maximum personal independence.

But such a policy needs people to carry it through. In the past gaps in staffing have traditionally been filled by nursing personnel, but the complex needs of the growing number of elderly people now filling the majority of wards in our hospitals are making increasing demands on nurses and there is little time to give the more individual patient-centred activity that many would like to do. Nor does the traditional pattern of ward organisation allow much opportunity for flexibility and elderly patients in long-stay wards are forced to fit into an arbitrary routine which has little relevance to life as they have known it, passing their days (and their lives) away, incarcerated in restrictive armchairs, inactive, bored, and increasingly dependent.

The need to prevent this type of situation and to find adequate help and above all continuity of helpers caused the Department of Geriatric Medicine at Edgware General Hospital to take positive action some thirteen years ago. The permitted establishments in professional manpower were stretched to their limit and voluntary workers, although helpful, could not afford to *give* their services as freely as

they were needed. Eventually a category of welfare aide was found
that ensured payment of a salary and was accountable to the
department's Administrator rather than being assigned to one specific
discipline, and thus the aide's role could be multi-functional.

An advertisement placed in the local press asking for part-time
help to enable elderly disabled people regain independence
produced overwhelming response, demonstrating the community's
goodwill and desire to help. No other qualification was required other
than the applicant should have a liking and concern for people and
a common-sense and practical approach, with a readiness to learn
and understand the special needs and problems of elderly patients.

Over the years, as financial resources have allowed, the number of
aides has increased and since their function is 'to help, to re-enable
people to live again as sentient sophisticated adults',[2] they became
known as 're-ablists'. They come from a variety of backgrounds, the
majority being married women with families growing up and each
has a strong desire to make some contribution by giving help where
it is needed most.

Much of their work takes place on the hospital wards working
closely with therapists and nursing staff. Daily they encourage
patients to wash, dress, walk, or if wheelchair patients, wheel
themselves to the lavatory and learn to manage there. In
conjunction with the occupational therapists, they help to organise
a wide variety of individual and group activities, both therapeutic
and recreational. Many have cars and can help with transport for
home visits with patient, remedial staff or social worker to meet
relatives and to work out problems in the home situation.
Patients can be taken out on shopping trips or longer outings and, on
discharge home or to residential accommodation, the patient
can frequently be taken by a re-ablist, which gives an invaluable
continuity link. Moreover, once home, patients can be visited on an
informal basis and this can be an acceptable way to maintain contact,
especially with elderly people living alone without supportive
relatives near at hand. In this way re-ablists act as the eyes and ears of
the hospital team and can report back any problems they may
encounter on a visit.

Perhaps the re-ablists' greatest value is that they have *time*. They
have not become swept up in pressures to complete tasks as are
nursing personnel, nor to deal with long lists of patients' treatments,
so frequently the case with remedial therapists. Although each day
needs to be structured, there is a built-in flexibility, so that re-ablists

have time to make contact with patients at a different level from the professional. They have time to listen and to talk and time, too, for all the small but important personal needs that tend to get overlooked on busy wards.

Although in 1971 the category of welfare aide was replaced by the now official Department of Health and Social Security grade of occupational therapy and physiotherapy helper accountable to the trained therapist, by now their interdisciplinary role had been firmly established. Any attempt at this stage to introduce professional demarcation lines was clearly impossible. In the field of geriatric medicine there is need for a great deal of overlap between the remedial professions, for the multiple physical, emotional and social needs of elderly patients can only be met by a therapeutic programme which avoids all unnecessary fragmentation.

Over the years, re-ablists have become an integral part of the Department of Geriatric Medicine's therapeutic community. Clearly this two-way experiment has not been without its problems. A great deal has been learned by all those involved and the learning process is a continuing one.

It is necessary that there should be flexibility with regard to working hours and it has always been made clear that domestic crisis and school holidays claim priority. Paradoxically, however, little time off is taken and such is the re-ablists' feeling of involvement and commitment that difficulties can usually be overcome and extra help given if it is needed.

Although members of the community find little difficulty in understanding the concept of a multidisciplinary worker, the re-ablist's role does tend to cause some perplexity for hospital personnel used to clear lines of demarcation between professional disciplines. This can be especially so in the case of nursing staff, because there can be a good deal of overlap between nurse and re-ablist in such basic activities as encouraging patients to wash and dress or in helping them to get to lavatory or commode.

Initially, too, nurses can feel resentment that re-ablists appear to work convenient part-time hours and there is often failure to understand that these hours could have been given to other part-time and probably more lucrative employment in some other field.

Of primary importance is the selection of appropriate personnel, for much depends upon the quality of people recruited. Inappropriate personalities — those for example who are authoritarian in their attitude and approach — can so easily upset the balance of an integrated team and this will have repercussive effects upon the patient. A probationary period is essential and this must be of adequate length to allow the new recruit to gain experience of the work involved and to give the trained therapist opportunity for careful observation of the individual's attitude and job performance.

Re-ablists participate in ward rounds, case conferences, staff meetings and study days, and visits are made to day centres, work centres, equipment exhibitions, hospices for the dying, wheelchair centres — the list is long. Within the Department of Geriatric Medicine itself, there is a constant exchange of ideas and discussion on problems of mutual concern by all members of the team and this provides for everyone a continual ongoing and educational experience. But perhaps of greatest value to the re-ablists is the day-to-day work on the wards, the relationship made with elderly people and the expanding and developing understanding of their needs and situation.

In-service training of a more structured and specific nature is organised at regular and frequent intervals. It is essential that for re-ablists' continued development, training must be ongoing. New recruits will need to understand the objectives, philosophy and function of the work of the department and their own particular role in helping to meet these objectives. Lines of communication need to be spelt out clearly so that the re-ablist knows whom to turn to in times of need. Training must be multi-disciplinary and all the disciplines involved should be prepared to contribute to these educational sessions from their own expertise and experience and this encourages professionals to keep up to date and to audit their own performance. Finally, as we have found, evaluation of training programmes is a necessary exercise, so that therapists and re-ablists together can identify gaps and weaknesses in the programme's content and ensure that it remains relevant to current needs.

## The Concept of an Added Dimension of Support For Patients in Hospital

The introduction of re-ablists to the Department of Geriatric Medicine at Edgware General Hospital has done much to enrich the lives of patients in the clinical and institutional world of hospital and to forge closer links with the community outside the hospital walls.

Retrospectively it has become apparent that an idea that arose originally from practical need has assumed value in its own right. The introduction of re-ablists has provided not a second class or substitute service for patients, but an added dimension of therapeutic support. Much of their value lies in the freshness and flexibility of their attitudes, unfettered by previous training; the sense of homeliness that they can generate; and the variety of skills and talents that they so frequently possess. Their role is a polyvalent or multidimensional one, bringing together under one title a range of activities and responsibilities and providing for each worker opportunity to make a unique contribution to total patient care and support.

## Expansion of This Concept for Patients at Home

In the project just described, re-ablists have been mainly deployed in a hospital setting, but their potential for providing this extra dimension of support for patients at home has unlimited possibilities.

Throughout the period of evolution of the re-ablist category, the Department of Geriatric Medicine has itself evolved, through a frenetic period of attempting to make hospital like home for its patients, to the realisation that this can never be. For if the objective of geriatric medicine is the prevention of institutional casualties, then to attempt solution of the medical and social crises of the elderly by admission to any form of institution is to risk producing long-term problems. Reliance on hospital or residential home facilities has been the professional and/or community response to dependency problems amongst the elderly and disabled for too long.

It is only relatively recently that we have begun to ask ourselves whether our highly specialised hospital-orientated system of health care is appropriate or even relevant in helping to meet the current needs of ill old people. Every piece of research in this direction has shown, almost without exception, that people who are supported in their own normal environment in times of illness are motivated more strongly to spontaneous recovery than those who are institutionalised.

For many years we have been merging our hospital resources as far as we can with those of the community. The suggestion that the National Health Service is more akin to stationing a fleet of ambulances at the foot of a cliff rather than providing a fence at the top has always been applicable in the tradition of geriatric medicine.

Clinically exciting crisis intervention has come naturally; prophylaxis or prevention, the more pedestrian and less obviously rewarding field of endeavour, has been slower to flourish.

For one of us the moment of truth came in a visit to Sweden in 1972, when visiting a superb hospital for old people. This hospital appeared to have all the architectural and clinical features and all the staffing requirements for which we had striven for so long. Despite all this, it was clear that the patients contained therein were no happier, nor was rehabilitation any faster, than in our own inferior conditions. Their patients, like ours, wished just as fervently to be in their own homes. This helped to give fresh impetus to our endeavours to maintain people at home.

An introduction to the French scheme of Hospital-at-Home, through an article by Freda Clarke,[3] together with the impending reorganisation of the Health Service in 1974, sealed our resolve to ensure that the elderly, in our particular community at least, should be offered *choice* in times of crisis, namely, whether to stay at home and receive all the services they would normally receive as occupants of hospital beds or to come into hospital in the accepted manner. To date in the United Kingdom the possibility of such a patient choice has been remote because the family doctor services, the social services, hospital services and voluntary services, despite numerous reorganisations, have remained as separate organisational entities. Theoretically, all work together to support such patient choice but practically, there is no co-ordinative structure to make this an attractive option for the professionals to select. If a member of one of the component services feels strongly that an old person should be maintained at home, then by painstaking endeavour over time, a supportive structure can be mobilised. At times of crisis, particularly during the unsocial hours of night, weekend or Bank Holiday, it is almost impossible to ensure enough continuous help at home to enable the sick elderly person to exercise choice, and admission to a hospital bed (if available) is usually the only solution.

Provision of a real Hospital-at-Home service hinges on a finely balanced structure of co-ordination and priority commitment between the services previously mentioned, with a task force ready on a 24-hour basis to be marshalled in the appropriate combination needed for individual situations. After the clinical diagnosis and assessment decisions have been taken, the first requirement in the home will usually be for the support of another sensible person to make the lone patient comfortable or to relieve an exhausted relative. Most family doctors say that there are very few episodes of illness in the elderly population they could not deal with in the home, if only the appropriate supporting services were easily contactable and instantly available.

The backbone of such a service must inevitably be the personnel involved, not only experienced, up-to-date, mature professionals, capable of assessing needs and inaugurating supportive programmes, but also the less highly trained person, the *aide-soignante* of France and the home health aide of the United States. In the United Kingdom at present we have the nursing auxiliary of the community nursing service and the home help of the social services. These are officially confined in definitive roles, the former to attend to the personal needs, the latter to the environmental needs of the elderly person. A meld of the two roles can easily be visualised in the person of a home re-ablist whose potential for providing this extra dimension and support for people at home has unlimited possibilities.

Of all the countries in the world the United Kingdom has probably the finest medium in the shape of health and social provision in which could flourish the whole variation of resources needed to support and maintain the ever-increasing numbers of elderly people in some degree of autonomy. Dr George L. Maddox went on record in a recent conference in Washington, DC, saying that it was his impression 'that the UK has very few health problems that adequate financing could not resolve satisfactorily'.[4]

Adequate financing is not the real problem. The basic difficulty is inflexible professional attitudes which fail to recognise that home care is the linchpin of health care delivery and that the main function of hospitals should be to provide skilled emergency treatment and technical services that can only be given in a centralised institutional setting.

Yet, professional attitudes are such that there is little confidence in such a concept, nor to date have effort and energy been directed to putting such a policy into practice. Naturally there also needs to be provision for the people who feel safer being treated in hospitals, but with the smoother meshing of domiciliary services, this need will inevitably decrease. Otherwise, for the majority, one can visualise hospitals being a 24-hour co-ordinating and resource centre, able to produce consultant medical, nursing and paramedical expertise, equipment of all kinds plus transport and, as a last resort, a back-up hospital bed. Inter- and cross-discipline education and communication can occur naturally and by design within such an organisation, and the professional and personal isolation felt by so many workers in the domiciliary fields will be mitigated. The growing confidence of the staff will flow over to the voluntary workers of family or neighbourhood and increased certainty that help will be forthcoming at time of need may short-circuit many breakdowns of a physical, social or emotional nature. Such breakdowns are very much the pattern of current crises, when an old person alone or a relative or neighbour has struggled too long with a heavy burden of handicap.

Fears have been expressed that providing services of this nature at home would prove an intolerable economic burden to already financially creaking services, but logically little of the funding would go into costly organisational structures or building maintenance. Currently 55-66 per cent of the National Health Service budget maintains the hospital services and structures. A dynamic redeployment of resources to focus at the point of impact, namely in the home, could predictably produce a very different scene for the elderly of the future to play a sturdier and more independent and contributory role in their final years. The implications for professional care-givers in such a context are profound.

## Division of Labour — Implications for the Professional

In any system of delegation where roles overlap and responsibilities normally assumed by the professional are shared with new kinds of workers, there tends to be for the professional a sense of unease and insecurity. Describing the study by Kaiser Permanente Medical Care System in Portland Oregon, on the training and use of multidisciplinary home health aides, Melissa Hardie refers to the following: 'While most medical care personnel can accept the multidisciplinary concept intellectually, their commitment can be less than total when the concept has to be implemented.'[5] Yet, as she goes on to say, these multidisciplinary workers (who were given training in social work, nursing and therapy skills) were able to provide over half the home care services which otherwise would have been provided by professionals. And the professionals themselves were utilised in training and in supervision. This raises many issues in terms of manpower, of costs and of interdisciplinary co-operation and has wide implications for professional care-givers.

A rapidly ageing population, the realisation that the vast majority of our patients today suffer from clinical conditions whose sequelae must be lived with, because their underlying cause cannot be cured, has had profound implications for the remedial professions. It is radically altering the traditional concept of therapy as we have known it. Today's therapist is less concerned with cure than with the restoration and maintenance of maximum personal capability, both physical and mental, for each patient, be he in hospital or in the community. Physiotherapy, for example, will involve assessment; the organisation of appropriate treatment programmes which frequently can be carried out by relatives, multidisciplinary aides, by volunteers or by nursing personnel; and in giving guidance help to all those concerned with the patient's support.

No less than 10 per cent of the world's population has some kind of disability. Speaking at the First European Symposium on 'Evaluation and Prospects of Physiotherapy',[6] Dr Helander of the World Health Organisation said that clearly it will not be possible to train 1.5 million physiotherapists in the developing countries, in order to equate manpower density to that of Western Europe now. In the industrialised countries of Europe and the rest of the world we have made people and patients dependent upon sophisticated technology and on highly trained professionals. Rehabilitation has developed as a highly specialised service and he suggests that if we are to meet the growing number of those in need then we must be prepared to simplify these services and to develop a less sophisticated kind of care that can be provided by the non-professional.

This does not rule out the need for the highly trained professional, but the value of such people will depend on whether they have learned to develop critical faculties which will equip them to move with the times. In the case of the remedial professions, we have to find effective measures to meet the implications of a changing situation. This means that we must reassess the priorities in terms of current need, evaluate present treatment procedures of questionable value, and be prepared to accept a new concept of ourselves as initiators, teachers and advisers. We have to acknowledge that our skills frequently lie in knowing what to do rather than doing it; that having assessed our patient's problems and planned a course of action, then these plans can be carried out as well or perhaps better by others. This will mean the creation of a system of shared and overlapping responsibility and interdependency, in which the helper has scope for personal initiative and opportunity to contribute by using her or his own personal skills and talents.

Faced with the multiple social and physical problems of elderly and disabled people, we professionals need help. Not as a means of propping up a collapsing service, nor as an attempt to deal with a crisis situation, but in order to provide that additional dimension for patients that we cannot of ourselves provide.

At Edgware General Hospital we have found from our own experience that the community contains an immense untapped potential. People are concerned and want to help. But the relationship between professional and assistant must be a creative one. To achieve this, we the professionals need a 'sturdy Ego'[7] — we need to be mature individuals capable of flexibility, imagination and self-knowledge, able to revalue present work patterns and we need to be 'aware that preoccupation with professional identity although understandable does not ensure the best service for the patient'.[8]

> The division of labour implies interaction: for it consists not in the sheer difference of one man's kind of work from that of another, but in the fact that the different tasks and accomplishments are part of a whole to whose product, all in some degree, contribute. And wholes in the human social realm as in the rest of the biological and physical realm, have their nature in interaction.[9]

### Appendix 1: Remedial Helpers — Job Description

*The Department of Geriatric Medicine, Edgware General Hospital*

### *General*

The term 'remedial helper' brings together under one title a wide range of characteristics, responsibilities and activities. It requires an individual who has been selected for a number of personal qualifications which will include temperamental stability, the capacity to relate to others with warmth and understanding, and a flexible and objective attitude towards her work.

The title is used to describe personnel who are initially unskilled, but who through a process of training and supervision are enabled to undertake specific tasks and thus to carry out that part of a treatment plan appropriate to the non-professional.

### *Remedial Helpers Working in the Department of Geriatric Medicine*

The objectives of any department of geriatric medicine is the restoration and maintenance of maximum personal capability, both physical and mental for each patient, be he in hospital or community. This will involve remedial therapists in:

(1)  Helping patients:
     (a)  to find a sense of volition and purpose;
     (b)  to regain and maintain maximum functional independence by encouraging practice in self-help activities.

(2)  Creating in the hospital situation a therapeutic and supportive environment where individual life-styles can be preserved and activities organised to provide stimulus and restore confidence and some measure of personal autonomy.

Remedial helpers will be expected to assist in carrying out these objectives in co-operation with professional members of the therapeutic team, sharing responsibility and having scope for personal initiative and opportunity to contribute.

*Job Title:*     Remedial Helper
*Department:*    Geriatric Medicine
*Hospitals:*     Edgware General Hospital, West Hendon Hospital,
                 Orme Lodge and Stanmore Cottage Hospital
*Organisation:*
*(a) Accountable to Superintendent Physiotherapist or Head Occupational Therapist* through senior physiotherapist or occupational therapist in association with:
(1)  occupational therapist
(2)  physiotherapists
(3)  nursing staff
(4)  remedial helper colleagues
(5)  speech therapists
(6)  social workers
(7)  medical staff
(8)  administrative staff
(9)  voluntary workers

*(b) Responsibilities*
(1)  Administrative: record-keeping; secretarial
(2)  Personal duties: a remedial helper
     (a)  is a member of a multi-disciplinary team sharing responsibilit'
          with other team members;

    (b)  understands the importance of maintaining confidentiality;

    (c)  recognises situations beyond her/his ability to handle and is able to report these appropriately;

    (d)  works with patients either individually or in groups using skills with which she/he is familiar, in (i) assisting in programmes of functional retraining by encouraging practice of self-help activities; (ii) helping to plan and organise therapeutic, recreational and work-orientated group activity;

    (e)  assists remedial therapists and social workers in carrying out home visits for the purpose of (i) patient assessment and/or resettlement at home; (ii) maintaining links with the department's patients residing in the community;

    (f)  participates in case conferences, seminars and other educational activities associated with the geriatric service.

*(c) Interview and Selection*

The Superintendent Physiotherapist and Head Occupational Therapist are jointly responsible for interviewing and selection of candidates and must ensure that each:

    (a)  fulfils a probationary period of three months before final appointment;

    (b)  receives in-service training and keeps a record of this.


### Appendix 2: Training of Helpers in Department of Geriatric Medicine

Effective rehabilitation in all its aspects needs a team approach. Thus training in basic principles of rehabilitation will be an interdisciplinary exercise.

*(1) Interview and Selection.* Care in interviewing and final selection is essential. Sufficient time must be given to this, and if possible applicants should be given opportunity for a brief tour of the department. The Superintendent Physiotherapist and Head Occupational Therapist are jointly responsible for interviewing and selection of candidates.

*(2) Probationary Period.* A preliminary trial period before final acceptance is very necessary and is helpful both to new recruit and to professional staff.

*(3) In-service Training.* Needs and policy will vary from hospital to

hospital. The majority of applicants will be married women, with domestic commitments, recruited mainly from the local community. Thus on-the-job or in-service type training would seem most practical and appropriate.

*(4) Duration of Training Programme.* An initial organised induction course of approximately three months would seem most satisfactory. Training will nevertheless be an ongoing process, regularly or on-demand booster training sessions continuing throughout the length of service.

### Contents of Training Programme

*(1) Orientation.* The emphasis here will be on orientation to the Department of Geriatric Medicine, but some preliminary description of the hospital as a whole should be given.

Many hospitals produce an information booklet and this can be helpful. So, too, is a map or plan of the hospital area.

New recruits will need to know briefly the location and function of the various departments within the hospital. An explanation of the accepted lines of authority will be necessary.

*Specific Orientation.* This will include:

(1) A description of the Department of Geriatric Medicine. Here a large map or chart will aid understanding.

(2) An explanation of the role and function of the personnel involved.

(3) Explanation of the aims and policy of the department. This will involve an appreciation of the particular needs of patients and an understanding of their special problems and situation.

(4) The place of the helper within the team.

(5) Ward etiquette and the special importance of maintaining confidentiality.

(6) Introduction of new recruit to all personnel and to fellow 'helpers'.

*(2) On-site Practical Training.* This will take place both on the hospital ward and in the rehabilitation department, and thus much of this instruction will overlap.

*Hospital Ward.* Here there can be help from nursing staff in learning simple procedures, such as giving bed-pans and urinals.

From paramedical staff, the emphasis will be on encouraging independence in personal activities and instruction will be given on all aspects of patient management.

The occupational therapists will give instruction on the organisation of group activities. Demonstration on the use of hoists, of bed cradles and of anti-pressure equipment, etc., will involve both nursing and therapy staff.

*Rehabilitation Department.* Demonstration and practical work here will include:

(1)   Activities and principles of basic independence:
    (a)   moving in bed, rolling on to the side, bridging;
    (b)   transfers;
    (c)   getting up from a chair and sitting down again;
    (d)   wheelchair management;
    (e)   walking with crutches, sticks and walking frames;
    (f)   management in the lavatory, dressing and feeding activities.
(2)   Instruction on:
    (a)   equipment and apparatus;
    (b)   wheelchair models, accessories and modifications;
    (c)   the management of calipers, below-knee brace and prostheses.
(3)   Methods of lifting.
(4)   The management of specific disability, such as 'strokes', multiple sclerosis, Parkinsonism, fractured femur, etc.

In addition to practical work, there will be talks and discussions on a variety of patient-related subjects by relevant personnel, e.g.
(a)   disorders of the special senses — speech, hearing and sight;
(b)   hospital hazards such as constipation, incontinence, dehydration, confusion, pressure sores;
(c)   patients: social backgrounds the role and needs of relatives and the function of community services.

The objectives of in-service training will be to ensure the development of each individual helper's maximum potential.

There will need to be regular feedback from the training sessions so that the content can be reviewed in the light of experience, in order that optimum effectiveness is maintained.

## Notes

1. Nancy T. Watts, 'Task Analysis and Division of Responsibility in Physical Therapy', *American Journal of Physical Therapy*, Vol.51, No.1 (1971).
2. Monnica C. Stewart, *My Brother's Keeper?* (London, Health Horizon, 1970).
3. Freda Clarke, *Hospital and Social Services Journal* (July 1973).
4. George L. Maddox, 'Research Developments and Implications' in *Care of the Elderly* (London, Academic Press; New York, Grunt and Stratton, 1977).
5. Melissa Hardie, 'You and Research', *Social Work Today*, Vol.7, No.8 (1976).
6. E. Helander, 'World Strategy for Disability Prevention and Rehabilitation', *World Health Organisation Chronicle*, Vol.30 (1976).
7. Nancy T. Watts, 'Task Analysis and Division of Responsibility in Physical Therapy'.
8. M.B. Hawker, 'Helpers/Aides Division of Labour', *Physiotherapy*, Vol.60, No.7 (1974).
9. E. Hughes, *Men and Their Work* (New York, The Free Press, 1958).

# 8 BIG FLEAS HAVE LITTLE FLEAS – NURSE PROFESSIONALISATION AND NURSING AUXILIARIES

Malcolm Johnson

As is so often the case in periods of change and uncertainty, it is possible to detect powerful paradoxes in the debate about the nature and content of modern nursing. Recent commentaries are frequently about, or prefaced by, historical accounts of the profession where leading figures like Florence Nightingale are reassessed. The persistent reader will soon become accustomed to rediscoveries of human frailty, self-advancement, passion, toughness, and even political ambition. These analyses – as we shall see later – are fierce in their search for features which either blemish or replace the sainted image of the lady of the lamp. The paradox is that in the face of historical toughening-up, there is an emergent cry which exhorts nurses to return to their traditional caring role at the bedside.

In one sense, this dialogue is the essence of this chapter, for I am concerned to try to illuminate the place of the least qualified practitioners of nursing in the process of professionalisation. In so doing it will be necessary not only to give some theoretical attention to the broader meanings and processes involved, but also to examine some of the new dimensions raised by restructuring within health care and the rise of feminism. Authority, policy involvement, role expansion, physician/nurse relations, male/female dominance patterns and the nature of required rewards are all amongst the topics under review. It may be that these items are flying round in the vortex of thrusting professionalisation and as such have a shape and meaning which can be examined.

Nursing has long attracted the title of 'profession', and its members have bathed in the reflected glory of professional status without possessing a number of the features essential to the establishment of that status. This ambivalent position appears not to have caused concern amongst rank-and-file nurses until the past few years. Despite this, the representative bodies have a long history of status battles both lost and won. So, whilst practical nursing has always been of a handmaidenly variety and at least formally under the control of physicians, bodies like the RCN and GNC have fought to establish the foundation of full professionalisation – autonomy.

Now, a new ideological element has to be taken into account. Nurses are conventionally female, and doctors male. Women's studies and the women's movement have not been slow to exploit the underlying theme of sexism in the medical scene. Yet concurrently with the establishment of this set of arguments, women attained equal proportions in the entry to British medical schools and the concepts of the nurse practitioner and physician's assistant have become working realities. Nurses have also joined doctors and administrators at every level and rank in the National Health Service as administrators and policy-makers. Ironically, nearly a third of these senior nurses are men.

Even at this stage it must be clear that no single mode of explanation or prescription will summarise the current situation. By taking professionalisation as the theme, we none the less have a back-cloth which takes account of both conceptual issues and pragmatic ones.

### Nursing and its Functions

When I first began to read the sociological nursing literature in the mid-sixties, the general argument about the subordinate position of women was only a latent theme. In the eyes of influential writers of the time, the conflicts were about whether nursing was a knowledge-based technical activity or one which specialised in tender loving care. This dichotomy led Sam Schulman to write about the mother surrogate role as a major contribution to medical care which no other agency was able to provide. Given that the constant attention, humane concern, body- and morale-maintaining activities and monitoring skills are all significant and valued contributions, the question was raised as to why nurses should want for more.

Much chided for his audacity and ten years older, Schulman[1] returned to his theme in the revised edition of Jaco's reader. Indeed, much of his later piece is devoted to recounting the strengthening of will amongst organised nurse opinion. Along with Hans Mauksch,[2] he notes the elements of change on the American scene. More graduates were (and still are) entering and seeking swift seniority in administration and management, whilst others pressed hard for the right to carry out technical procedures which matched their superior intellectual and practical training. They documented the beginnings of a stratification of nursing with a substantial university-educated élite crossing the gap between the subordinate nurse and the autonomous doctor. But patients have other needs than venepuncture, intravenous infusions and the rest. Traditional nursing skills continue to be called for, creating a new gap between the nurse at the bedside and the nurse with her bag of equipment.

Mauksch's paper, 'Nursing: Churning for a change?'[3] sums up in its title alone the unrest on the American nursing scene in the late sixties. It could equally be applied to the British situation of today. Following the major upheavals of Salmon,[4] reorganisation and the renewed introspection over Briggs,[5] industrial relations initiatives and stronger demands for women's rights, a similar turmoil exists. However, it would be wrong to suggest that the two national scenes are merely replicas of each other, with Britain dragging along a few years behind. The university-trained nurse is a new entrant to the British hospital and associated with that situation is the relative lateness of the arrival of a respectable academic base for nursing studies. By contrast, American nursing has accommodated many thousands of graduates from undergraduate and master's degree programmes since the turn of the century.

Britain's later entry into the academic field provides a good indication of the different bases upon which professionalism has been pursued here. In this century the nurse, both in hospital and in the community, has held a position of respect in society which has, in some senses, transcended the class system. A special kind of social reward, which Weber called status honour, has been accorded to her both as a just reward for the social value of her work and as a substitute for a proper financial return. Moreover, nursing retained its social acceptability through the continued recruitment of girls from upper-class backgrounds whose families found it a suitable prelude to marriage, or a wholesome career for those who might fail in the marriage market.

What has happened on both sides of the Atlantic is that a more assertive attitude amongst nurses at all levels has challenged both the profession's structural status *vis-à-vis* medicine and health care and its own social order. Thus organised nursing faces both the enemy without and the enemy within. Its fate in its striving for full professional status is therefore in the short run hampered by its inability to act as a unified body.

Unity and the creation of a base of its own technical knowledge are not new objectives in British nursing. Brian Abel-Smith[6] tells of the acrimonious disputes which took place about the proper direction of nursing when the College of Nursing was founded in 1916, and this was only one of many earlier attempts to organise nurses. Later attempts to secure registration reinforced the élitist elements which had already entered the activities of the College. College membership was restricted to those whose training had been completed, according to detailed requirements in general hospitals or infirmaries with at least 250 beds. Such rules excluded many, particularly mental nurses, children's nurses and male nurses. The situation was further exacerbated by the requirements for registration when they were instituted.

Rival groups of nurses, like the Professional Union of Trained Nurses (formed in 1919) sought unity through other channels, but the divisions between hospital- and community-based nurses have early origins which none of these developments succeeded in repairing. The primary goals of the various bodies seem in restrospect to be less distinct than debates at the time suggest. Educational standards, professional status and better monetary rewards seem to have figured, in differing degrees, in them all. And to draw an even more acute parallel with contemporary development, the College set up a fund to establish a university chair in nursing in 1918. Soon after, they were successful in mounting diploma courses at the Universities of Leeds and London.

An historical review of divisions in nursing is not the primary concern of this chapter, but some indications of the roots of present-day circumstances are essential. Before returning to the contemporary world it is worth spending a little time assessing the growing number of statements which reconstruct the myths of early nursing history. The very phenomenon – legitimate as it is an historical exercise – raises interesting questions about the motives and the timing of their production.

Elvi Whittaker and Virginia Olesen[7] raise many of the issues which have become part of the feminist approach in a paper descriptively titled 'The Faces of Florence Nightingale: Functions of the Heroine Legend in an Occupational Sub-Culture'. They are eager to point out that any biography can be seen from a variety of standpoints and that any historical figure can be seen to have had several 'faces' or images. This is clearly true of Miss Nightingale. Her few months serving the soldiers in the Crimea have served history well, though they were a very small part of her nursing career. None the less they encapsulate her image as heroine. Whittaker and Olesen suggest that this image is no more than a fictionalised elaboration of the truth.

They go on to say that 'her main concerns were not with the wounded *per se* but rather with the higher levels of administration and with manipulation of the Cabinet at home.'

The woman of intellect and authority, the woman who was a nuisance to politicians and governments, the woman who reputedly had many lovers, are all lost. The romanticised version fitted neatly with a period of romanticism and humanitarianism. In addition, she represented what Whittaker and Olesen call the 'safe sacrifice'. Thus they conclude that

> Upon further examination of the popular face of Florence Nightingale, it becomes clear that it represents those aspects of femininity which are deemed culturally desirable. The historical face, on the other hand, presents her with characteristics tinged with masculinity, aggression and divorcement from the home and family aspects of femininity. These latter aspects are not entirely acceptable for women in our society, and hence appear to remain the province of history rather than become part of the popular image.

In a more recent paper on nurse practitioners and the problems they face in achieving the status and authority to practise independently, Bonnie Bullough[8] returns to the theme of the over-feminised image of nursing. She examines the barriers facing that section of nursing which has expanded its role into the physician's territory. These she claims are rooted in legal restraints promulgated long ago on the basis of the past subordination of women and, in particular, of nurses in their occupational role. In seeking explanations for this situation, she turns the spotlight on Florence Nightingale, who 'even though she helped create a work role for women which took them outside of the home, the nursing role was shaped in a completely traditional manner and the accepted interaction patterns of the sexes were not disturbed.'

Rewriting history in this way is an essential by-product of social change and those who do it are not just destroying myths for the sake of discrediting revered figures. Nightingale's reputation seems secure, despite the retrospective wishes that she had been a reformer rather than a conserver of the social values of her day. She has merely become the personified focus of an emergent woman-power which is bound to have profound influences on nursing, both for those women who provide care and those who receive it. As Carol Brown[9] points out, over 85 per cent of all (US) health service and hospital workers are women, but most of the work is controlled by men. Equally, there is a developing awareness amongst women as consumers of health care that medicine as practised through the male medical model is frequently unacceptable, damaging or both.

As far as some writers on nursing are concerned, any issue within the occupation of nursing must be seen as part of a disabling history and a sustained sexist ideology within organised medical care. These constraints clearly affect the professionalisation process to which we now turn and influence the way in which innovators and leading thinkers conceive those who function as nurses but who have no credentials to testify to their skills – auxiliaries.

### Nursing – A Profession?

Since Flexner[10] conducted his celebrated analyses of the characteristics of professions from 1910 onwards, there has grown up a vast literature within sociology. Much effort has been expended on selecting out the vital features which together transform an occupation into a profession. However, no one has satisfactorily compiled such a list of attributes. There has been surprisingly little agreement amongst the lists and it is not possible to point to a synthetic compilation which ties the definition down.[11] A further review of the problems is not required here, but a few observations about the deficiencies which have hampered nurse professionalisation are necessary.

In order to avoid a check-list approach we will use a summary statement at the very commencement of Eliot Friedson's major analysis of the medical profession:[12]

> This book presents extended analysis of a profession. As its title implies, emphasis is on both sides of the meaning of the word – 'profession' as a special kind of occupation, and 'profession' as an avowal of a promise. As I shall try to show. . .it is useful to think of a profession as an occupation which has assumed a dominant position in a division of labour, so that it gains control over the determination of the substance of its own work. Unlike most occupations it is autonomous or self-directing. The occupation sustains this special status by its persuasive profession of the extraordinary trustworthiness of its members. The trustworthiness it professes naturally includes ethicality and also knowledgeable skill.

Certain elements of this package of characteristics are demonstrably present within nursing in general — though not present for all categories of nurse. Thus we can reasonably talk of nurses being a special occupation which has engendered a trustworthiness and respect for its basis in knowledgeable skill. Yet these things can only be said in general, so long as nursing is seen as those practitioners who are qualified SRN or its equivalent. Can we really say the same for SENs or for the large army of mainly untrained nurses who represent more than half of the nurses at the bedside? No such case has ever seriously been made and the wide dispersion of skills and education levels has been a constant concern to those who have sought to attract to nursing the additional benefits which accrue to occupations which have functional autonomy.

The first serious attempts to unify nursing for this purpose were made prior to the Nurse Registration Act of 1919. The College of Nursing at that time was anxious to achieve some sort of uniformity which would encompass selection and training, leading to a position where there could be public guarantees of competence in areas peculiar to, and preferably exclusive to, nursing. Their hoped-for model for the registering body — The General Nursing Council — was the medical equivalent (the GMC) with all its authority and prestige. But as Celia Davies[13] points out, there was neither clarity of thought nor unanimity from the nursing bodies and the resulting Act left many residual anomalies and unresolved issues. Not least of these were the terms and conditions for registration itself.

Immediately after the First World War a vocal group amongst nursing leaders had set themselves the task of achieving the twin objectives of uniformity and autonomy. Neither have been fully achieved sixty years later, although there are areas of uniformity and pockets of autonomy. Common standards in training have occurred, but the specialist divisions have adopted educational and internal political positions which make uniformity almost impossible in reality, though the common base of registration made it at least possible. In line with these specialist splits comes the distribution of autonomy. Some have had a large measure of control over their work for many years and these are notably forms of nursing which take place outside hospitals and therefore away from surveillance, or which have thus established such a tradition. Midwifery and health visiting represent the relatively autonomous groups. Clinical assistants who carry out functions previously performed by physicians represent the new group of independent practitioners. Their common characteristics are to be found in their post-SRN status and the length of the training involved. However, none of them has truly escaped from medical direction.

The continuing uncertainties of even these élite members of the nursing community is highlighted by Jean Donnison[14] in her comments on the Briggs Committee recommendations. In commenting on the Committee's proposal for a joint regulatory body, she suggests that a Standing Committee on midwifery will not assuage the fears of midwives about their special status. In particular, 'they have fears that they will henceforth be classed, officially as well as unofficially, with nurses *rather than as practitioners in their own right'* (emphasis added). These same concerns, born of female challenges to the present medical system, are expressed in the American setting with rather more force and purpose.[15]

Clinical assistants are still few in number in Britain, having been introduced experimentally in only a few hospitals. In the USA, where they are much more common, there is a potential threat and a potential set of opportunities associated with the parallel development of physicians' assistants. These intermediate practitioners, with less than the full medical training, represent another route to the territory of the clinical assistant which is not in any way confined to trained nurses. The threat, therefore, is whether they can continue to maintain separate identities and retain for nursing a stake in intermediate medical practice. The potentiality is that the development may lead to a continuum of health science degrees which will allow nurses to qualify as physicians' assistants and then as doctors.[16]

Whichever turn of events comes about, the prospects for uniformity and autonomy look bleak. Without uniformity it looks distinctly more likely that some nurses will be able to fill the new spaces in any newly created hierarchy of clinical practitioners.

Only in the area of management can we confidently talk of true autonomy. Since Salmon was implemented in Britain in the late sixties and more especially since reorganisation of the NHS in 1974, there has been an exponential growth in nursing administrators at every level from the ward up to DHSS. It is now widely accepted that the Salmon system was introduced for the good of nursing as an occupational group without a proper career structure, rather than as a system for improving patient care. From its introduction we gained a rigid hierarchy of management which filled the void between nursing sister and matron (or her assistant). Yet for all its managerial bias and the much-vaunted principle of sapiential authority, it is very much a top-down system with accountability of a high order.

At the higher levels of post-reorganisation times, where there has been a greater functional split, autonomy has been handed out to those nurses who found themselves in planning, personnel and the like. Perhaps most important, nurses have now achieved what the Royal College of Nursing sought at the time the NHS was set up – equal status and representation with administrators and doctors at all levels. But the price of this explosion of management is the divorce of all but a few senior nurses from clinical work. Many commentators have signalled the detrimental effects this has had on the coherence of nurses as a group, for it has put them into an us-and-them situation which denies any unity which might derive from common training and interests.[17]

Thus the three main categories of nurses who have moved closest to professional status are those upon whose skills the whole reputation of nursing was forged; but they are divided amongst themselves and quite distinct from the main body of people who provide the bulk of nursing care.

## Big Fleas have Little Fleas. . .

So far we have paid little attention to nursing auxiliaries. Our concerns have been with those who carry the weight of nursing prestige. But the hospital patient, whose view of nursing is coloured by the professionalised image projected over the past six decades, is likely to be treated by an unqualified person. In writing of changes in nursing a British Chief Nursing Officer very recently wrote of American nursing:

> The head nurse of the ward (whose range of responsibility resembles that of our ward sister) spends the major proportion of her day at the nursing station directing and organising; her actual personal contact with patients in the area is extremely limited. The nurse who actually nurses the patient is often the male or female with only basic training (if any at all).
>
> In theory these nursing assistants and 'practical nurses' are supervised by the registered nurses, but in the majority of hospitals the pattern has now been accepted where this supervision is minimal if existent at all. Sadly the trend has led to a situation where the nursing care in an average hospital can be of an extremely low standard.[18]

His assessment extended to the British scene in similar vein, criticising
the over-emphasis on management and advocating higher priority for
patient care.

When then ought we to expect of the nursing auxiliary? Hockey[19]
reminds us of the many definitions and terms which surround the
subject but points out that their primary function, as untrained or
partially trained personnel, is to assist the trained nurse in her work.
The Royal College of Nursing offered the following as its definition:

> Nursing personnel able to perform specific tasks related to patient
> care that require considerably less use of judgement. They should
> be able to relate well to patients and carry out dependably under
> supervision, the tasks for which they have been trained.[20]

This definition seems to beg more questions than it answers. What is
meant by specific tasks ?  Is there a range of identifiable tasks which are
suitable? What sort of judgements might an auxiliary make or not
make? What is an acceptable standard of supervision? These all seem
very relevant questions in the light of claims that many of these
individuals are working in a manner which endangers patients, the
more so when one examines Hockey's own findings. In answer to a
question about the amount of responsibility given to auxiliaries, an
overwhelming proportion of nurses and administrators
who worked with them felt it was 'just about right'. Significantly
the only noticeable dissent from this view came from staff nurses and
midwives, whose supervisory contact would be the closest. Almost
one in five of them felt too much responsibility was given.[21]

The stratification we noted earlier seems to have reached a stage
where some urgent repair work is necessary and some careful thinking
about the performance of basic nursing tasks is essential. Traditionally
the apprentice nurse in her various guises has had the privilege of the
'dirty work'. Sluices, vomit removal, faeces and domestic cleaning
were all part of learning to be a nurse. Indeed, cleaning out the
sluice room was in times past a common punishment for juniors who
were caught in the worthless act of talking to patients. Both sluice
rooms and disapproval of direct communication with patients are now
much less in evidence. In their place, the learner and her companion
in labour, the auxiliary, are delegated such nobler tasks as walking
elderly patients to the lavatory or changing the sheets of the
incontinent. Yet paradoxically much of the essential human contact

which provides the therapeutic drive of nursing is to be found in these unlikely circumstances.

In response to being given the dirty work, the nurse in training either leaves, becoming another unexplained statistic in the nurse wastage figures,[22] or faces up to her lot as the price she must pay in order to qualify. The auxiliary, with no credentials to gain and no career structure to climb, faces different alternatives. She too might resign and seek other work, but the auxiliary is almost by definition an unqualified person whose marketability is low. In the present climate of unemployment and economic restraint, she is more likely to stick to her post in mounting frustration. Her position as a hired hand at the bottom of the pile in nursing is the one which offers least in the way of status and improved monetary rewards.

Part of my argument has been that the unqualified nurse is in many ways the person carrying out the most vital of the nursing duties. She has constant contact with patients and is frequently the one to whom they turn both for comfort and information. Julius Roth, in his study of TB patients in the early sixties,[23] showed how the lowest level of nursing personnel provided the best (if not the most reliable) sources of information upon which to base their own time-tabling. This is reinforced by many recent studies and specifically in relation to details of diagnosis, prognosis and for conditions which carry communications taboos.[24] As a result, there is a real basis of job satisfaction to be derived from patient contact, patient gratitude and their projection of higher capabilities than their training warrants. But these tangible positives must be seen within an overall work context which takes into account relations with senior colleagues and the system of formal rewards.

Research for the Briggs Committee found that some qualified nurses had already decided against seeking promotion on the basis of their unhappiness with the new managerialism. Conflict between clinical nurses and their managerial superiors has been brewing since Salmon and has not been assuaged either by the growth of post-graduate clinical training or the emergence of nurse practitioners. This mood of unrest is predictably not confined to career-blocked trained nurses. The untrained nurse who finds her orders coming from ever-loftier quarters has come to despise many of the directives for their inappropriateness. At the same time, she is resentful of the lack of support in the daily routine of tasks which too often take her beyond her true competence.

The situation stretches the rules of deference to their limits. The totally subordinate position of the auxiliary demands a deference to many levels of authority; but in this climate we might speculate about its authenticity. Howard Newby[25] has examined the literature on deference and feels that it fails to come to terms with the many discrepancies in expected and real situations because it does not distinguish clearly enough between behaviour, attitudes and socially held beliefs. Thus deferential behaviour should not be taken as confirmation of a deferential attitude. It may merely be a useful mode of achieving some desirable end like gaining time off to go to a wedding or keeping the pressure of surveillance down to a minimum.

This is a mode of behaviour that Goffman[26] calls 'impression management', and one which people use when they are 'on stage'. The metaphor is of a social drama where the term 'on stage' refers, let us say, to conversations auxiliaries have with the sister in her office, but who then go 'off stage' as they return to their work. A good deal of deferential behaviour is ritualised and habitual, like the soldier's salute or the addressing of superiors by their rank (sister, doctor, etc.). Consequently it cannot be a reasonable guide to the *attitudes* it represents. If deference is to be meaningful, the behaviour must faithfully represent an attitude, and not just be a piece of impression management. Therefore, Newby suggests that 'real' deference occurs only where there is a congruence of behaviour and attitudes, but that deferential behaviour which denies the underlying attitude is calculative and thus essentially non-deferential.

There seems to be great potential for calculative behaviour in the role of the nursing auxiliary who has acquired skills and understanding through experience. In recent years she will have witnessed industrial action amongst her trained colleagues which served to widen the gap between the trained and untrained. But she too has become increasingly unionised, as Tom Manson[27] indicates. The auxiliary, increasingly in the front line of nursing care, lives in a nursing world preoccupied with education, research and management. She sees the occupation of which she is a part moving away from sustained patient contact in pursuit of other more status-oriented goals. Thus a rift is occurring between those who provide the front-line patient care and those who control their work. How long will it be before the thin bonds of deference are strained beyond their elasticity?

## Conclusions

Historically, nursing has existed within a highly ordered and hierarchical system of medical care. It has conventionally been subordinate both as an occupational entity and because of its almost exclusively female composition. In pursuit of its professional goals, nursing has constantly attempted to create a unity which could lift the occupation as a body of well-trained women into the full professional status of functional autonomy. In order to do this the representative bodies have attempted to create autonomy in selected areas of their work. To date we can see autonomy of a sort in the work of a new breed of post-graduate clinical nurses and through managerialism.

On the whole attempts at creating a replica of the medical professional model have failed badly, though there have been some useful spin-offs. Despite its demise, this sequence of events has led inexorably to a massive concern with high standards of training and research rooted in universities. Respectability and a unique body of knowledge have been the twin objectives. This, we have argued, has caused splits within the occupation of nursing which are most marked as they relate to auxiliaries.

Feminism as a powerful ideology has accompanied and reinforced the thrust to autonomy. This has brought in its train an anxiety to rewrite the publicly known history of nursing. Femininity is no longer the keyword of nursing[28] and thus the feminine models have to be reconstructed. In a world of female emancipation and legally protected equality of opportunity, this women's work is gaining attributes which can bring it in competition with the male-dominated profession of medicine. However, we cannot conclude that these manoeuvres have been concluded with decisive effect. Nursing remains without the essential formal professional characteristics.

Perhaps the greatest stumbling block to professional elevation is the vast range of work which goes on under the nursing rubric. Nursing auxiliaries are not only numerous, they carry out work of an undeniably important kind with little or no training. This very situation is a matter of rising concern, for the social distance being created between the qualified and unqualified practitioner is likely to lead to a militant response from below. Authority must command respect, and there are some grounds for believing that the workers on the ground floor of nursing are breaking out of their traditional deference.

Whilst economic circumstances preclude the implementation of the Briggs Report recommendations, their concern to unify nursing through the creation of a continuum of training, skills and specialisms is a sound one. The present élitist approach will inevitably cause deep divisions which even the most ardent of professionalisers has wanted to avoid. Diversity is a characteristic of nursing which is to be cherished. Unity does not mean uniformity. So if the goal of professional status is to continue to be high on the nursing agenda, may I suggest that the words of a part contemporary of Florence Nightingale's, Augustus De Morgan, be ever borne in mind:

Great fleas have little fleas upon their backs to bite 'em
And little fleas have lesser fleas, and so ad infinitum.[29]

## Notes

1. Sam Schulman, 'Basic Functional Roles in Nursing: Mother Surrogate and Healer' in E.G. Jaco (ed.), *Patients, Physicians and Illness* (New York, Free Press, 1958); Sam Schulman, 'Mother Surrogate: After a Decade' in E.G. Jaco (ed.), ibid., second edition, 1972.
2. Hans Mauksch, 'The Organisational Context of Nursing Practice' in F. Davis (ed.), *The Nursing Profession, Five Sociological Essays* (New York, Wiley, 1966).
3. Hans Mauksch, 'Nursing: Churning for a Change' in H.E. Freeman, S. Levine and L.G. Reeder (eds.), *Handbook of Medical Sociology* (Englewood Cliffs, NJ, Prentice-Hall, second edition, 1972).
4. *Report of the Committee on Senior Nursing Staff Structure* (the Salmon Report), Ministry of Health (London, HMSO, 1966).
5. *Report of the Committee on Nursing* (the Briggs Report), Cmnd 5115 (London, HMSO, 1972).
6. Brian Abel-Smith, *A History of the Nursing Profession* (London, Heinemann, 1960).
7. Elvi Whittaker and Virginia Olesen, 'The Faces of Florence Nightingale: Functions of the Heroine Legend in an Occupational Subculture', *Human Organization*, Vol.23, No.2 (1964).
8. B. Bullough, 'Barriers to the Nurse Practitioner Movement: Problems of Women in a Woman's Field', *International Journal of Health Services*, Vol.5, No.2 (1975).
9. Carol A. Brown, 'Women Workers in the Health Service Industry', *International Journal of Health Services*, Vol.5, No.2, (1975).
10. A. Flexner, 'Is Social Work a Profession?' *School and Society*, Vol.1 (1915), pp.901-11.
11. G. Millerson, *The Qualifying Associations: A Study in Professionalisation* (London, Routledge and Kegan Paul, 1964).
12. E. Freidson, *Profession of Medicine, A Study of the Sociology of Applied Knowledge* (New York, Dodd and Mead, 1975).
13. Celia Davies, 'Constraints on the Development of Occupations', unpublished paper presented to the BSA Medical Sociology Group Conference, September 19

14. J. Donnison, *Midwives and Medical Men* (London, Heinemann, 1977).
15. Barbara Ehrenreich and Deidre English, *Witches, Midwives and Nurses, a History of Women Healers,* Glass Mountain Pamphlet No.1 (New York, Feminist Press, 1974).
16. Ann Suter Ford, *The Physician's Assistant, a National and Local Analysis* (New York, Praeger, 1975).
17. Cf. J.W. Paulley, 'Is it too late to scrap Salmon?' *Nursing Times,* Vol.67 (1971), pp.212-13, and Michael Carpenter, 'The New Managerialism and Professionalism in Nursing' in Margaret Stacey *et al.* (eds.), *Health and the Division of Labour* (London, Croom Helm, 1977).
18. T. Kerrane, 'Challenge of Changing Patterns of Nursing', *Health and Social Service Journal,* Vol.37 (2 September 1977).
19. L. Hockey, *Women in Nursing: A Descriptive Study* (London, Hodder and Stoughton, 1976).
20. World Health Organisation, *Report of the Expert Committee on Nursing* (Geneva, 1966).
21. L. Hockey, op.cit., p.171.
22. See G. Mercer and C. Mould, *An Investigation into the Level and Character of Labour Turnover amongst Trained Nurses,* Final Report to DHSS, 1976 (unpublished).
23. Julius Roth, *Timetables: Structuring the Passage of Time in Hospital and Other Careers* (Indianapolis, Bobbs-Merrill, 1963).
24. J. MacIntosh, *Communication and Awareness in a Cancer Ward* (London, Croom Helm, 1977).
25. Howard Newby, 'The Deferential Dialectic', *Comparative Studies in History and Society,* Vol.17, No.2 (April 1975).
26. Erving Goffman, 'The Nature of Deference and Demeanour' in his *Interaction Ritual* (Harmondsworth, Penguin University Books, 1972).
27. Tom Manson, 'Management, the Professions and the Unions: A Social Analysis of Change in the NHS' (unpublished).
28. Victoria Wilson, 'An analysis of Femininity in Nursing', *American Behavioural Scientist,* Vol.15, No.2 (1971).
29. Augustus De Morgan, *A Budget of Paradoxes* (1872), p.377.

# PART TWO:
# THE INTERNATIONAL BACKGROUND

# 1 AUSTRIA    Miss F. Dittrich

The professional groups in the Austrian nursing services are: registered general nurse, registered sick children's and infants' nurse, registered psychiatric nurse, registered midwife. Auxiliary personnel, and their minimum training hours, are the following:

'Stationsgehilfen' – undertaking a very limited number of general auxiliary duties. Minimum hours of theoretical tuition: 185.

'Operationsgehilfen' – helping only in operating theatres and first-aid rooms. Minimum hours: 135.

'Sanitätsgehilfen' – helping with patients' transport. Minimum hours: 135.

'Desinfektionsgehilfen' – helping with duties in relation to disinfection. Minimum hours: 135.

Legally, no personnel without an official designation may be employed. The current trend is to reduce auxiliary employment. Auxiliary personnel may only work in hospitals and residential homes. There are no domiciliary auxiliaries.

Training is specific to the specialty, e.g. the auxiliary for operating theatres learns about personal hygiene, disinfection and sterilisation; simple instruments and their use; first aid and bandaging; principles of X-rays and ray hazards; principles of social insurance, indemnity insurance and legal rights; principles of hospital administration. All other trainings have similar specialty emphases.

# 2 BELGIUM Mrs A. De Smet Simoens

The Royal Decree No.78 of 10 November 1967, relating to the art of healing, the exercise of related professions and the medical commissions (subsequently modified by the law of 20 December 1974) laid down the principle that, as from November 1967, nursing could be practised in Belgium by those who possess the diploma or title of graduate nurse (refers to both female and male), the certificate ('brevet') or title of nurse and the certificate or title of assistant nurse and who

121

had their titles visa'd by the competent authorities.

The statutory requirements that hospitals and their services have to fulfil provide that the qualified nursing staff should be in charge of nursing care, but that they should be assisted by auxiliary nursing personnel numerous enough to administer all the necessary care.

The latter group is very heterogeneous and is referred to in the hospital as 'unskilled personnel'. When drafting the strength of the personnel in a hospital, the ratio generally aimed at is 70 per cent qualified personnel and 30 per cent unqualified personnel.

There is no statute in Belgium that imposes a uniform training scheme on the auxiliary staff. At present this staff is largely composed of persons with a schooling in health care leading to the certificate of 'children's nurse' or 'home and sanitary help' (three years of study; pupils are aged between 15 and 18). Others had a more limited training in first aid provided by the Belgian Red Cross. Still others received an in-service training in various departments.

It has become customary for hospital managements to guide this heterogeneous group with theoretical and practical lessons, which they organise at their own initiative, most often with the help of the qualified nursing staff. This training aims primarily at teaching the auxiliary staff members some basic skills. Providing them with a theoretical background is only the secondary goal.

The various tasks for which this particular category is eligible are neither clearly defined nor regulated. Nor are the functions of this group legally protected. In order to compensate for the shortage of nurses, the Minister of Public Health has on several occasions recommended hospitals to replace nursing staff by other personnel to carry out non-nursing or non-attending duties.

In practice, auxiliary personnel have up to now been charged with administering hygienic care to patients, with 'hostel' services and with various domestic duties. The enforcement of the above-mentioned law will restrict the activity of these persons in the near future to the last two duties, excluding all nursing treatment. Yet the law also stipulates that — as a temporary measure — the auxiliary staff who have been employed in a hospital, or with a physician or a dentist, for at least three years are allowed to carry on their duties under the same conditions as those that apply to nurses. The anxiety to administer quality nursing care has led the health authorities to urge all auxiliary staff already employed to qualify as a nurse and to give an impetus to this training within the framework of the paid educational leave scheme. Many hospitals organise courses and provide facilities for their unqualified staff so that they can prepare for the examinations of the Central Examining Board leading to a nursing qualification. The professional bodies of nurses, too, have taken similar initiatives in order to attain that goal.

## 3 CANADA Sister Mary Lucy Power

In Canada there is only one category of trained nurse — the Registered Nurse (RN). Each province has its own licensing body, the provincial registered nurses' association, which must approve the credentials of all nurses applying for work within the province. Nurses are trained in a variety of situations — University Schools of Nursing, which give a Bachelor of Nursing as well as the RN, three-year Schools of Nursing based on two years of theory and one year of practical training (rapidly disappearing) and two-year Community College Schools of Nursing. All of these students write a common Canadian registered nurse examination to acquire their Registered Nurse diploma.

There is in Canada an auxiliary nursing group called Certified Nursing Assistants. These are also provincially controlled and have a specified training period (usually 10 months). Curriculum varies from province to province, although the objective generally is to prepare a person to provide basic nursing care under the direction of a nurse or qualified medical practitioner and to assist the registered nurse in the care of acutely ill patients. Although there is a Canadian examination for this classification, not all provinces take advantage of it at present. There is across the country a wide variety of policies as to duties, responsibilities and capabilities of these assistants.

There is then another category which has a variety of titles — untrained nursing assistants, aides, etc., who are usually trained on the job, have a lesser degree of responsibility and do not write an examination.

## 4 DENMARK Mrs I. Gyde-Petersen

Within the personnel groups in the Danish hospitals two groups are employed in the nursing and care of the patients, nurses and nursing assistants. At present, approximately 28,000 nurses and 36,000 nursing assistants are working in Denmark — mainly in the hospitals and the rest in social welfare (in nursing homes, looking after the aged and chronic sick and so on). These figures include both full-time and part-time workers.

*The nurses* are trained in schools attached to the larger hospitals. The course of instruction extends over 3½ years, with theoretical and practical work in different hospital wards and departments. This training is an authorised statutory training.

*The nursing assistants* are trained at schools run by the hospital service. Their basic training consists of 3 months' theoretical instruction (300 hours) and 9 months' practical work in hospitals. This training was approved by the Ministry of the Interior, the employers and the employees in 1973. Earlier, this training consisted of 8 months (approved in 1960). The normal field of activity for the nursing assistant is clearly defined in a government circular, which also defines the fields of responsibility for this personnel group. The Ministry has also approved a plan for compulsory in-service training — consisting of 98 hours' theory — for all nursing assistants to bring their knowledge up to date. In addition to that, the hospitals must work out introductory and instruction programmes for specific fields.

Special training for nursing assistants working in the operating rooms and theatres has been approved also. This training consists of 23 weeks' theoretical instruction and practical work. Nursing assistants in nursing homes for aged and chronic sick patients receive a 12 months' theoretical and practical training.

The training of nurses, nursing assistants, as well as many other hospital staff, such as therapists, laboratory assistants and senior catering staff, is laid down and supervised by a special committee under the Ministry of the Interior (Council for Training of the Health Services Personnel) with representatives of several ministries, as well as the National Health Service and the Association of County Councils. Professional training of hospital personnel is carried out on a uniform basis all over the country, and all nursing and patient care services in Denmark are only carried out by trained personnel. The 'volunteer' principle is unknown.

Tenure, salaries and working conditions for nursing assistants are the same over the whole country. This has arisen through working agreements between the organisation representing the personnel and the hospital authorities (the Association of County Councils,

Copenhagen Municipality and the National Government).

In Denmark about 2,300 nurses and 4,000 nursing assistants annually are taken on and trained. Nurses as well as nursing assistants have their own national organisations and their own pension funds.

## 5 FEDERAL REPUBLIC OF GERMANY
Oberin W.V. Poncet,

In the Federal Republic of Germany there are two categories of trained nurses:

(1) Krankenschwestern/-pfleger: three-year general nurse training
Kinderkrankenschwestern/-pfleger: three-year children's nurse training

(2) Krankenpflegehelferinnen/-helfer: one-year general nurse training

The standard of nurse training schools, the minimum entrance standard for students and the content of training is set by government legislation. The candidate who successfully passes the state finals is licensed by the state authorities to practise nursing under the professional title respectively of,

Krankenschwester/-pfleger
Kinderkrankenschwester/-pfleger
Krankenpflegehelferin/-helfer

It is therefore the professional title which is protected by law, whereas nursing itself is not restricted to the professional nursing staff.

In addition to the above-mentioned nursing staff and the learners (student nurses and pupil nurses) of each category, there is a third group of nursing care workers which are referred to in statistics as 'other nursing personnel without state examination'. At present, this group constitutes approximately 20 per cent of the nursing work-force (excluding learners). Though it is not yet shown in the statistics, there may be a present decline in usage of this group.

About 75 per cent of these 'other nursing personnel' are still employed in general and psychiatric hospitals. The remainder work in old peoples' homes, etc.

Nursing personnel in the Federal Republic of Germany, including West Berlin, on 31 December 1974 (Stat. Bundesamt nach Verl. Kohlhammer, DKZ 8/76):

| | |
|---|---:|
| Krankenschwestern/-pfleger | 150,344 |
| Kinderkrankenschwestern/-pfleger | 21,058 |
| Krankenpflegeschülerinnen/-schüler<br>(student nurses general nursing) | 44,851 |
| Kinderkrankenpflegeschülerinnen<br>(student nurses children nursing) | 10,343 |
| Krankenpflegehelferinnen/-helfer | 39,097 |
| Schülerinnen/Schüler Krankenpflegehilfe<br>(pupil nurses) | 9,146 |
| Other nursing personnel without state examination | 51,530 |

Of the 'other nursing personnel', many have been attending a nurse aid course (SH). These courses are financed by the government and are run by the Red Cross, the Maltese Association and the Association of St John. They last four weeks and comprise 100 hours of theoretical lessons, given by doctors and nurses, followed by 100 hours' practical work under supervision in general hospitals, and a final examination. Some 200,000 girls and women – no men – have attended these courses in the last 25 years. SH are supposed to help with basic nursing tasks in their own families, in the neighbourhood and in emergencies. The SH courses are not intended to train SH for skilled nursing duties in hospitals. Nevertheless, when applying for a hospital job, in recent years the SH usually has been preferred to applicants without a SH course. The SH working in hospital was at all times legally considered as 'other nursing personnel' and also paid on the same basis.

With the growing number of 'other nursing personnel' in hospitals, the DKG (German Hospital Society) in 1965 made a recommendation for a one-year training scheme as a possibility for untrained staff to qualify on a not too demanding level. This recommendation was taken up by a number of hospitals and in 1965, with the amendment of nursing legislation, a one-year training programme with a state examination for the 'Krankenpflegehelferin' was introduced officially for the first time.

Because of the growing number of 'Krankenschwestern' with three years' training, untrained staff, including SH and even the

'Krankenpflegehelferin', find it increasingly difficult to get jobs in the hospital.

# 6 FINLAND Mrs P. Lyytikäinen

In Finland it is only nurses (2½ years), psychiatric attendants (1½ years) and auxiliary nurses (1 year) who receive education for ordinary nursing. In addition to this, we have several smaller groups of educated nursing subgroups (e.g. x-ray technicians). The main working groups at ward level are nurses, auxiliary nurses, children's nurses and hospital assistants. The ratio of nurses, auxiliary nurses and hospital assistants in wards of general hospitals is as follows: nurses 35-45 per cent, auxiliary nurses 35-42 per cent and hospital assistants 19-25 per cent. Variety in ratios depends on the character of work in the ward. The hospital assistants are not counted as nursing staff. Their primary tasks in wards consist of cleaning and maintenance of equipment. Recently, however, some tasks connected with nursing have been given to this group, e.g. bed-making and helping at meals. No nation-wide general education has been organised for this assistant group. However, every hospital attempts to give in-service training, which contains theory of cleaning, working positions and general hygiene. About 70 per cent of the hospital assistants have received this kind of training.

The education of auxiliary nurses lasts two academic terms (20 weeks) and consists of both theoretical and practical studies in ordinary nursing (in various specialties). Moreover, lectures are given in basic biological and in social subjects. The tasks of the auxiliary nurses consist mainly of basic nursing care but, depending on the character and staff situation in the ward, the work can also include service tasks and even such nursing tasks for which basic education is not required. In-service training is the method by which this staff learn to carry out such tasks for which no lessons are given.

Recently there have been lively discussions about prolonging the educational term of auxiliary nurses. The matter has not been resolved yet, because we are now preparing a wider reform of medium-level education in Finland which will also concern health care staff.

Health care institutes, which include general hospitals, mental hospitals and tuberculosis sanatoria, do not generally use untrained staff; it only happens in most urgent situations when qualified staff are not available. However, some institutes of social care, e.g. those for mental defectives and old peoples' homes, use untrained staff for nursing tasks to some extent. Nursing students are not counted in Finland as a labour force.

Number of positions in 1976

|  | Hospitals | Primary Care | Total |
|---|---|---|---|
| Nurses | 14,442 | 6,919 | 21,361 |
| Matrons | 413 | 410 | 823 |
| Laboratory and X-ray technicians | 1,643 | 841 | 2,484 |
| Auxiliary nurses | 5,184 | 2,700 | 7,884 |
| Children's nurses | 1,479 | 364 | 1,843 |
| Hospital assistants | 6,454 | 1,363 | 4,817 |
| Health centre assistants |  | 2,083 |  |

The above figures should be multiplied by approximately 1.2-1.3 to arrive at the number of staff needed (persons) to undertake all tasks. During the last few years we have had difficulties getting enough nurses for health care duties. The number of students trained as auxiliary nurses has been increased. Simultaneously, a few positions of nurses have been changed to those of auxiliary nurses. This kind of change forces a consideration of the division of labour in nursing. The national five-year plan for health care also urges hospitals to adjust the division of labour. This adjustment would make it easier to calculate the need for staff positions and their training.

## 7  FRANCE Miss M.L. Badouaille

In France there are two categories of nurse: the state registered nurse, who is qualified to do general nursing, and the mental nurse, who is trained to care for patients with mental illnesses. In both cases, the diploma is granted by the Ministry of Health and Social Security after the student has passed a final examination. The training courses are different in content but identical in duration — 28 months.

The following statistics may be of interest:

|  | State Registered Nurses | Authorised Nurses | Mental Nurses | Total |
|---|---|---|---|---|
| 1974 | 122,417 | 20,790 | 39,459 | 182,666 |
| 1976 | 138,616 | 21,036 | 44,054 | 203,706 |

There has, therefore, been a clear increase in numbers. In 1974, of the 122,417 state registered nurses, 68,678 were employed in general hospitals (excluding old people's homes). The remainder were either working outside the hospitals or teaching in the basic or post-basic nurse training schools. The mental nurses are similarly distributed.

The nursing team receives help mainly from staff called *aides-soignantes*. In 1974 these numbered 94,311, about three-quarters of them working in the public hospitals. Their training lasts for 12 months and successful students obtain an *aide-soignante* diploma.

In some institutions working in maternal and child welfare (ante- and post-natal clinics, crèches, day nurseries, short-term nurseries, in shopping centres, blocks of flats, etc.), paediatrics and maternity departments in hospitals, we also find nursery nurse helpers, classified as staff who work under complete supervision. Their training is 12 months long, including holidays. Student nurses, although they are extremely useful, are not considered as supportive staff. In 1974 there were 45,341 students training in schools for their general diploma; in 1976, this number was 56,752. There is, therefore, a very clear increase in the number of nurses in training. The same is true for the psychiatric sector. This increase is linked partly to the growth in the number of schools of nursing (in 1974, there were 285 schools for general training; in 1976, 328; also in 1976, there were 142 centres training mental nurses).

The nursing situation, although still difficult, has clearly started on the road to improvement. Within about a year, the length of the course will be extended from 28 months to three years. The legal definition of the nurse is being reviewed so that she will no longer be considered, in official documents, simply as someone who carries out the orders of the doctor but as a professional with her own area of autonomy.

The public health sector is developing. In order to foster interdisciplinary work, there are plans for the future to train all the managers in the health professions in the same schools or institutes. Continuing education is gaining ground.

Many problems have still to be solved, however, which include:

the financing of our schools and of the individual nurse in training; the shortage of nurse teachers; the distribution of tasks/duties between nurses and *aides-soignantes;* the strengthening of the nursing service; the development of nursing research.


## 8  UNITED KINGDOM Mrs M. Hardie


In the UK two categories of trained nurses are licensed to practise. These are the state registered nurse (SRN) and the state enrolled nurse (SEN).* The licensing authorities are the General Nursing Council (GNC) for England and Wales, the GNC for Scotland and the Northern Ireland Council for Nurses and Midwives. In addition to these two categories of nurses, two other large groups of nursing care workers are employed by the health authorities: learners — student and pupil nurses training for the Register and the Roll as above — and an indeterminate group referred to in government statistics as 'other nursing staff'. The latter personnel group encompasses workers who are variously called auxiliaries, aides, assistants or attendants. Whether or not these various titles should carry the prefix 'nursing' raises controversies, but increasingly in the last decade these employees have been centralised within the nursing establishment and under nursing management. At present within the National Health Services — hospital and community — these employees constitute approximately 30 per cent of the nursing work-force and in 1972 a government report, the *Report of the Committee on Nursing* (Chairman: Asa Briggs), predicted that by 1980 the proportion will have reached one-third.

National Health Service: Manpower Summary (1973)

| | |
|---|---|
| Hospital nursing staff: | |
| Registered nurses | 108,373 |
| Student nurses | 60,450 |
| Enrolled nurses | 55,551 |
| Pupil nurses | 27,657 |
| Other nurses | 105,764 |
| Community nursing staff: | |
| Home nurses | 12,170 |
| Health visitors | 7,688 |
| Other general nursing staff | 5,814 |

* Designations of these categories in Scotland are Registered General Nurse (RGN) and Enrolled Nurse (EN).

A wide spectrum of policies and practices affect the employment of these nursing auxiliaries. While government departments have issued memoranda of guidance on the duties and responsibilities of nursing auxiliaries to employing health authorities, there is no legislation covering these and no prescribed instruction for the job. Traditionally, auxiliaries have been prepared by on-the-job training at the discretion of the local hospital or community nursing service and inevitably the instruction is oriented to the particular worker's responsibilities rather than based on a background of theoretical studies. While having its advantages, inherent in this method are the difficulties associated with flexibility, change of employment and the understanding of an individual's employment by other health workers. There is professional disagreement as to the extent of their duties. These duties may vary considerably, both within one health authority and nationally. Appointments are made on the basis of interviews and letters of recommendation and, in a very few cases, on simple literacy tests. From that point on, the nursing auxiliary's work can vary from some basic nursing skills, such as bed-making and maintenance of equipment, to dealing with complex interpersonal and technical situations which arise in the nursing care environment.

Some health authorities offer formal introductory courses of instruction in nursing care and general orientation to the hospital or community centre from which the employee will work. Increasingly 'in-service training officers' are seeking to organise and in some cases centralise courses of instruction, study days, etc. to provide continuing support to this staff group. Hardie and Hockey, in their study, 'The Nursing Auxiliary in the National Health Service' (UK, 1976-7), indicate the wide range of variation in how these responsibilities are undertaken by the local health authorities.

Among the issues raised by this employment pattern in the United Kingdom are: allocation of duties/division of labour between nursing grades; appropriate training for the tasks/duties allocated; the nature of professional supervision and implications for the training of professional nurses; resource allocation both for the training of nursing workers and future employment ratios; deployment of nursing auxiliaries within hospital and community systems in regard to medical and nursing care specialisation.

# 9  NETHERLANDS Miss Hanneke M. Th. van Maanen

Category III Nursing Personnel, as defined by the International Council
of Nurses, is

> Nursing Personnel able to perform specific tasks related to *patient*
> care that require considerably *less use of judgement.* They should
> be able to relate well to *patients* and carry out dependably, under
> supervision, the tasks for which they have been trained (WHO
> Expert Committee on Nursing, 1966).

According to this definition, in which I emphasised the words that are
specifically related to health care and to the level of education of the
worker, the Netherlands do not employ, neither do they promote, the
employment of auxiliaries. However, the Netherlands recognise several
categories of other workers in and outside the health care system.

As manpower-planning and staffing problems are giving cause for
concern in several countries of Europe and in some parts of the USA,
it may be of interest to know how a small country like Holland managed
to keep auxiliaries outside its health care institutions. Before giving a
brief explanation about these categories of other workers, some insight
will be given in nursing personnel staffing in the Dutch hospitals.

In the Netherlands two categories of nurses are qualified to
practise:

(1)  The professional nurse – verpleegkundige, defined by ICN
as Category I.
(2)  The practical nurse – ziekenverzorgende, defined by ICN as
Category II.

The supervision over and control of nursing education and practice
is the responsibility of the Ministry of Public Health and Environment.
The Nursing Act governing *nursing education* dates from 1921 and has
been amended at various times and is going to be revised. This Act
introduced registers for general nurses and psychiatric nurses. Since
the establishment of nursing education programmes for practical
nurses, this group has also been registered on graduation.

There is no legislation, however, regulating professional *nursing
practice,* but in view of the nurse's increasing responsibility and
accountability an urgent need for enactment is widely accepted.

The draft act is expected to reach Parliament shortly.

The Dutch hospitals are staffed by nurses and student nurses. The majority of the student nurses are educated in hospital schools of nursing and are at the same time employed as 'workers' by their training hospital. This is an unfavourable situation as educational goals are of secondary importance to nursing service. The first responsibility is to staff the wards with an adequate number of people. Nursing services are, however, increasingly interested in nursing education as a means of safeguarding the quality of patient care.

The practical (student) nurses are in the first place employed by the nursing homes, as their training is mainly focused on basic nursing care, care for the chronically ill and rehabilitation. The education for practical nurses is offered in schools affiliated with nursing homes. Because of some staffing problems in the general and psychiatric hospitals, some of these institutions have employed practical nurses as well. Although this employment is definitely not promoted by the Ministry of Health and Environment, the reality had to be faced. In order to protect the practical nurse against assignments for which she has not been adequately prepared, guidelines for employment have been provided to the hospitals. The practical nurse can be assigned to the care of the chronically ill (including patients with rheumatism), geriatric and rehabilitation patients.

Reasons why auxiliaries have not been employed in the Dutch hospitals:

(1) The Ministry of Health and Environment and the Dutch Hospital Association are not in favour of employing unqualified people in the hospitals.

(2) The wards are staffed with nurses and student nurses. Student nurses as working force are covering some tasks that in other countries may be assigned to other categories of personnel, e.g. bed-making, bed baths, mouth care. Basic physical care is regarded as essential for nursing.

(3) Housekeepers have taken over all kinds of tasks that used to be performed by student nurses, e.g. cleaning of wards.

(4) Departments like central supply, bed-cleaning service, centralised food and diet distribution have lightened the domestic work-load of nurses.

(5) The Central Committee for Hospital Fees (COZ) is controlling the hospital expenses and accordingly regulating by certain financial

mechanisms the planning of personnel in hospitals, including nursing services. Within the limitations of the available and permitted budget, a balance has to be found in higher and lower qualified staff. This decision is made at management level. As the proportion between nurses and student nurses is officially 40:60 (although in reality it is coming closer to 45:55), in order to guarantee safe care there is no tendency to increase the number of students or to consider the employment of low- or untrained personnel.

## 10  NORWAY Miss E. Kristiansen

Nursing auxiliaries are defined here as 'personnel assistant to the qualified registered nurse in the delivery of nursing services'.

By a nursing auxiliary is therefore understood any helper to the qualified registered nurse in her delivery of nursing services to patients/clients.

Two groups of auxiliaries can be defined.

(1) Personnel with formal training as nursing assistants.
(2) Personnel without any formal training as nursing assistants.
(Ward assistants whose main function is cleaning of the ward are not defined as *nursing* auxiliaries and will not be dealt with here.)

According to accepted policies for budgeting and staffing for the nursing services, nursing auxiliaries are in Norway supposed to have completed a formal training programme of 10-12 months. These auxiliaries do possess a registration as qualified nursing auxiliaries. (These may be compared to the registered practical nurse.)

The training has from the early sixties been given in special programmes either in independent schools for nursing auxiliaries, programmes affiliated to hospitals, or in vocational school programmes. The programme is approved by the Department of Health and Social Services and consists of theory components of a total of 415 class hours and practice components of a total of 28 weeks. Applicants have to be 18 years of age on admission and have completed a minimum of 9 years of general education. Many adult learners do complete the programmes successfully and are later stable auxiliary workers in the health care system. The programmes prepare nursing auxiliaries for the following fields of nursing:

(1) general nursing care, mainly focused on somatic aspects;
(2) psychiatric nursing;
(3) care of children;
(4) care of mentally retarded.

Specially trained auxiliary personnel to other fields, as for example geriatrics, may be coming soon.

A new proposition regarding the education of personnel to the health and social services did pass Parliament in the spring of 1977. According to this, it is expected that the training of auxiliary personnel will be done through programmes integrated in what is called continuing education for students aged 16-18 (secondary school, junior high school). Details on curriculum content and organisation are not yet clarified. Neither is it clear whether these programmes will produce auxiliaries at different functional levels.

One special concern to the Norwegian Nurses' Association (NNA) with regard to the new educational system for auxiliaries is the low age of the auxiliaries during their schooling and immediately after graduation. NNA has required that the majority of the professional subjects and all the practical training should be given in the last of the three years of continuing education. Then most of the students are in their eighteenth year. The previous two years should be devoted to general education.

In spite of the present policy of having all nursing auxiliaries prepared for this function through training programmes, auxiliary personnel without any relevant training are working in the nursing team in most institutions. Three different categories can be defined:

(1) Untrained auxiliaries employed because no formal qualification was required for the position. The qualifications were expected to be developed through work experience. These will be found mostly in mental hospitals, nursing homes and some other long-term institutions. Auxiliaries belonging to this category have usually now been in their positions for many years and account for a large number of the nursing personnel in some institutions of the kind mentioned above. Most institutions are now working on this situation.

(2) Untrained auxiliaries employed because of shortage of trained personnel. Most of these are also found in long-term institutions (somatic, geriatric, psychiatric).

(3) Students in need of earning credits for admittance to medical schools, schools for physiotherapy, medical technicians, work

therapists, nursing, etc. These may go into regular positions as nursing auxiliaries for four months to one year, or they may go into special trainee positions with a smaller salary (at present 1800 N. kr. a month, which amounts to about one-half of the monthly salary of a nursing auxiliary).

The table shows the numbers of qualified nurses, qualified nursing auxiliaries and auxiliaries without relevant training in Norway in December 1975 and their allocation in some categories of somatic institutions and within these institutions.

The Number of Qualified Registered Nurses* and Midwives, Qualified Nursing Auxiliaries and Nursing Auxiliaries Without Formal Training in Norway in December 1975

| | | | |
|---|---|---|---|
| Qualified registered nurses and midwives | | 14,335 | 67 per cent full-time  33 per cent part-time |
| Qualified nursing auxiliaries  7.768 | 75 per cent full-time  25 per cent part-time | | |
| Nursing auxiliaries without formal qualifications  5.732 | 67 per cent full-time  33 per cent part-time | 13,500 | 72 per cent full-time  28 per cent part-time |
| Nursing personnel total | | 27,835 | |

*Qualified registered nurses include nurse specialists, anesthesiology, X-ray, operating room nurses, nursing administrative, etc.

Source: *Health Statistics 1975,* Central Bureau of Statistics of Norway (Oslo, 1977), ISBN 82-537-0714-2

Nurse staffing in institutions and primary health care is presently given much attention. In question is both the total number of nursing personnel, as well as the type of personnel needed and the number of auxiliary personnel to the number of qualified registered nurses.

It is recognised as important that the ratio of auxiliaries to registered qualified nurses is kept proportional to each other in a way which allows each of the two groups to take on the responsibilities for which they are prepared. It is further seen as very important that every patient should have a registered qualified nurse as his primary nurse who is working directly with the patient and is responsible for his care. Auxiliaries should be used as assistants in this work.

We are hoping for and working towards the time when resources we need to deliver safe and growth-promoting care will be made available through budgeting policies as well as educational policies.

## 11 PORTUGAL

Background information on the auxiliary in the Portuguese nursing services has been incorporated with the case paper delivered on this topic. See 'Auxiliary Nursing Personnel in Portugal — Evolution of the Situation and Trends', p.166.

## 12 SPAIN Mr C. Cerquella

Major changes have occurred and are presently occurring within the Spanish nursing profession. A brief background summary will clarify these changes.

Before 1953, there were three types of professional nurse: 'practicantes' — male nurses, on the whole, who worked as medical assistants, female nurses and midwives. 'Practicantes', generally male, though females were allowed, trained for three years at university, for which entry requirements were four General Certificates of Education (GCE). Both female nurses and midwives trained for two years at training schools attached to universities.

In 1954, these three professional bodies united under the name of Ayudantes Tecnicos Sanitarios (ATS). This did not, however, resolve the Spanish nursing problem. Female nurses, now required to do three years' training in residence, paying for their own course, were actually used as cheap labour. Alternatively, the male nurses went to university for their lectures and practised with little or no supervision. On completion of training, they registered in different nursing councils, females in the Female General Nursing Council and males in the Male Council. Most female nurses work in hospitals and male nurses in private practice.

To specialise, the registered general nurse must then complete a two-year post-graduate course, in his free time and at his own expense. The specialties are: obstetrics, psychiatry, physiotherapy, paediatrics, chiropody, laboratory, X-ray, health visiting and occupational health. There is an Advanced College of Nursing in Madrid, where nurse teachers and nurse administrators are trained. Since insufficient numbers can be handled there, the same course is offered also at Barcelona, Bilbao, Pamplona and in the Canary Islands.

Previously there had been many untrained nurses in hospital and therefore the six-month courses were instituted. These, however, did not appear to prepare workers sufficiently. In 1974 the Ministry of Education ordered a two-year course with entry requirements of three ordinary level GCEs.

The last two years have seen many discussions on improving standards of nursing care. There has been much unhappiness in the profession about the domination of nursing policies by medical doctors. It has been felt necessary to fight for the rights of nursing as a profession. Papers have been prepared by the General Nursing Council and the Advanced College of Nursing on improving educational standards. Helpful to us was a paper on Spanish nursing given by Miss Dorothy Hall, Regional Nursing Officer of WHO (Europe). This campaign has culminated in new legislation placing basic nursing education at university level. Minimum requirements will be four GCEs at ordinary level and three advanced, as for any other degree. At the close of training, registration will be in one unified General Nursing Council. The new University Nursing School begins in September 1977 and will cover three academic years (September-June). Those schools training student nurses at present which cannot meet the Ministry of Education requirements will become Level II (SEN equivalent) schools, or will be closed down.

In summary, only a part of what is wanted has been achieved. The majority of nursing education still lies in the hands of medical doctors. Until we have nurses with nursing education degrees, the same patterns will continue.

University Training for Professional Nurses

| | |
|---|---|
| Accepted: | Three-year course leading to Diploma in Nursing Thesis at the end of training. |
| Not Yet Accepted: | Following the above course, a two-year training leading to the degree of nursing, in specialties, education and administration. Thesis at the end of programme. |
| | Following the above course, a two-year doctorate degree in nursing, in specialties, education and administration. |

Practical Nurses and Technicians Training

Already Accepted:    Two-year course leading to 'Auxiliar de Clinica' (SEN equivalent). Entry requirement: 3 GCEs.

Two-year course leading to technician's high school certificate, in laboratory, X-ray, etc.

## 13 SWEDEN Miss I. Johnsson

### 1. The Nursing Auxiliary in Sweden

A survey covering all kinds of medical personnel is made yearly in Sweden. At the end of 1974 there were 47,800 *active* registered nurses and nurse midwives and 620 midwives. The total number of active nursing personnel, excluding personnel at institutions for the mentally retarded, amounted to 129,500.[1]

| | |
|---|---|
| Nurses (registered) | 47,800 |
| Midwives (registered) | 620 |
| Nursing personnel (practical nurses and nursing aides) at somatic hospitals | 67,530 |
| Nursing personnel at psychiatric hospitals | 13,550 |
| | 129,500 |

Nursing care in Sweden has for many years been partly carried out by auxiliary nursing staff working under the supervision of registered nurses. In the 1950s schemes were instituted in large cities to provide some training for these auxiliary workers.

One of the consequences of the rapid expansion of the health services in recent years was a lack of registered nurses. In 1959 a government committee[2] was appointed to investigate how nursing work was and could be distributed among nursing personnel. The committee was empowered to recommend which tasks could be transferred from registered nurses to auxiliary nursing personnel and to outline schemes of education for new categories of nursing personnel. The report of the committee was published in 1961 and since then an education is available for practical nurses and nursing aides which is in accordance with the tasks allotted to them. The practical nurse is legally responsible – in exercising her duties – in relation to her education.

The development of psychiatric care with possibilities of new treatments of psychiatric patients made it necessary to look into the 'personnel situation' of the psychiatric hospitals. In the year 1959 a government committee[3] started an investigation and presented in 1965 a rather detailed report about the organisation of personnel for psychiatric hospitals, including proposals about the education of this nursing personnel. An education was then established and the mental nurse became legally responsible.

The curricula, developed as a result from these reports and later modified, are applied in all schools in the country, where the education of practical nurses, mental nurses and nursing aides takes place. The education is at present drawn up within the framework of the general school system (upper secondary school).

This year the government has initiated a new investigation about the personnel structure of the health service. It can be presumed that this investigation will cover more categories of nursing personnel than the above-mentioned and that the results will be used to adjust the education of health personnel to present needs.

### Notes

1. Allmän hälso- och sjukvård 1974, Sveriges officiella statistik.
2. Arbetsuppgifter och utbildning för viss sjukvårds-personal, SOU 1962:4.
3. Mentalsjukhusens personalorganisation del 1 och 2, SOU 1963:24 och 1965:50.

### 2. Training the Nursing Auxiliary Ms B. Pettersson and Mrs W. Gavelin

In Sweden there is a rather high *differentiation of staff* in hospitals and other health institutions and the various categories receive training in accordance with the duties allotted to them.

The county councils in Sweden are training most of the hospital personnel in their own schools of nursing (excluding physicians and training for teaching and administration), and it is possible to choose between several approaches to professional training.

For *general hospital nursing* and *for geriatric care* the training schemes for nursing auxiliaries cover 23 weeks or 8 weeks. Further training to the rank of enrolled nurse is then available within these branches of the health services. Enrolled nurses in general hospital wards, operating rooms or out-patient units may proceed to registered nurse training. This course covers only three terms, thus taking into account their previously acquired knowledge (the length of general basic training for nurses is five terms).

Here we give two examples of training courses:

## 1. Basic Training for Nursing Auxiliaries (Aides)

*Requirements for admission:* Applicants should as a rule be 18 years of age, have school leaving certificate and be in good health.

The *length of the course* is 23 weeks (see Table 1).

*Functions after training:* Nursing auxiliaries (aides) perform nursing duties requiring less skill than the work of enrolled nurses. They may be assigned to such duties as bed-making, bathing and general hygienic care of patients, care of hospital equipment, serving meals and generally attending to the patients' comfort.

## 2. Training of Enrolled Nurses for Hospital Wards, Operating and Out-Patient Units

*Requirements for admission*: Applicants must have a certificate from basic training for nursing auxiliaries (aides) and at least two years of approved service as nursing auxiliary (aide).

The *length of the course* is 32 weeks (see Table 2).

*Functions after training:* The enrolled nurses assist in the general care and treatment of hospital patients. The importance of the enrolled nurses in the medical team has steadily increased. Enrolled nurses now perform many of the less complex nursing duties and thus free the registered nurses for more skilled and specialised work.

Table 1: Curriculum for Basic Training of Nursing Auxiliary Aide

|  | Average Number of Hours per Week | | |
| --- | --- | --- | --- |
|  | Period 1 Theory 5 weeks | Period 2 Practice 16 weeks | Period 3 Theory 2 weeks |
| (1) Practical instruction |  | 42 |  |
| (2) Theory of patient care: |  |  |  |
| (a) orientation about training programme | 2 |  | 6 |
| (b) principles of patient care | 13 |  | 11 |
| (3) Anatomy and physiology | 7 |  |  |
| (4) Hygiene | 6 |  | 7 |
| (5) Diseases and their treatment | 4 |  | 4 |
| (6) Psychology | 2 |  | 4 |
| (7) Social medicine | 1 |  | 5 |
| (8) Physical training | 2 |  | 2 |
| TOTAL | 37 | 42 | 39 |

The practical instruction is given during eight weeks in long-stay or similar wards and during eight weeks in primarily surgical units.

Table 2: Curriculum for Training of Enrolled Nurses for General Hospital Wards, Out-Patient Units and Operating Rooms

| | Average Number of Hours per Week | | |
|---|---|---|---|
| | Period 1 Theory 6 weeks | Period 2 Practice 24 weeks | Period 3 Theory 2 weeks |
| (1) Practical instruction | | 42 | |
| (2) Theory of patient care: | | | |
| (a) orientation about training programme | 2 | | 2 |
| (b) principles of patient care | 9 | | 7 |
| (3) Anatomy and physiology | 5 | | |
| (4) Hygiene | 7 | | 5 |
| (5) Diseases and their treatment | 4 | | 6 |
| (6) Nutrition | 1 | | 2 |
| (7) Pharmacology | 3 | | 4 |
| (8) Psychology | 2 | | 3 |
| (9) Social medicine | 2 | | 6 |
| (10) Physical training | 2 | | 2 |
| TOTAL | 37 | 42 | 37 |

The practical instruction is given during eight weeks in medical wards, eight weeks in surgical wards, four weeks in surgical out-patient or operating units and four weeks in other out-patient unit (of student's choice) or psychiatric ward.

## 14 SWITZERLAND Miss M. Hofer

In Switzerland two categories of trained nurses are licensed to practise. The are the registered nurse and the practical nurse. While the registered nurse is trained for 3 to 4 years, the practical nurse receives a training of 1½ to 2 yea The licensing authority for both categories of nurses is the Swiss Red Cross, which was entrusted with the responsibility for the training of the professional nursing personnel by the Swiss Federal Government.

In addition to these two categories of trained nurses and the learners for these professions, there are two categories of nursing auxiliary workers: the trained nursing auxiliary and the untrained nursing auxiliary. They are both members of the nursing team. While there are no numbers for the untrained nursing auxiliaries available, up to now about 4,500 persons have received a 1-year-training as nursing auxiliaries.

The training is given in a recognised school for nursing auxiliaries in hospitals with a minimum of 50 beds. The training comprises between 190 and 210 hours of theory. From the beginning, the nursing auxiliaries are integrated into the hospital ward. At the end of the training they must pass an examination which includes nursing auxiliary work, functioning of the human body, household work in the hospital and a subject of their own choice (e.g. first aid, technical service). On successful completion, they receive a certificate which is jointly issued by the responsible cantonal authority and the Swiss Conference of the Cantonal Directors of Public Health Affairs. Their field of activity includes the following duties:

— bathing of patients
— bed-making
— transport of patients to other hospital departments
— prevention of bed sores
— distribution of meals, feeding, preparation of tube-feeding
— preparation and application of dressings (plasters, poultices, etc.)
— preparation and application of electronic blankets or ice-bags
— administration of steam inhalations
— use of the thermometer
— recording of certain items in the nursing care plan (e.g. amount of fluid)
— performance of household duties attached to nursing (e.g. washing up of tea-cups, cleaning of lockers and beds, disinfection of material)
— maintenance of equipment
— aid in changing bedridden patients, in getting people up, in walking with patients
— observation of patients and informing the nurse in charge of these observations

As can be seen from the duties enumerated, the activities of the trained nursing auxiliaries are mostly located in the hospital. Community nursing is not yet as far developed as it is in the United Kingdom.

In addition to these trained nursing auxiliaries a large number of untrained nursing auxiliaries (aides) work in the hospital. They are prepared, if at all, at the discretion of the local hospital by an in-service training. In some hospitals they are given one to two theoretical lessons a week or they may have a special introductory programme of a week or two.

The range of duties they perform varies according to the type of hospital. In the nursing homes, the nursing auxiliaries may be in charge during night duties, while this is usually not the case in the general hospitals.

For both categories of nursing auxiliaries, this work may sometimes serve as a preparation for professional nursing training. About one-fifth of the trained nursing auxiliaries take up another nursing training later on. This gives to the profession an opportunity to test the suitability of a person for nursing.

The first schools for training of nursing auxiliaries were devised in about 1957. During the years of extreme shortage of nursing personnel, these usually well-trained people proved to be a great help on the wards. Nowadays the capabilities of each of the four categories of nursing personnel (registered nurse, practical nurse, trained nursing auxiliaries, aides) must be closely identified. Only this guarantees an economic assignment of labour.

# PART THREE: CASE PAPERS

# 1 THE CONSEQUENCES FOR NURSING WORK OF AN EXPLICIT DEFINITION OF THE TERM 'PATIENT'

## Stephen Cang (England)

Definitions are unpopular. The reasons for this are simple: either the definition is inadequate, in which case it causes misunderstanding and irritation, purporting to clarify but serving in fact only to confuse; or else it really does bite, in which case it demands some realignment of perceptions and thinking. So either way it is tough going. But at least the attempt to construct adequate definitions may help to diminish the confusion which besets so many working situations, where questions of who should be doing what, for whom, under what conditions, for what reward compared with whom, and with what freedom of action, are by and large consigned with a sigh and the expressed belief that it will all come out in the wash, a quaint English expression conveying the universal human wish that trouble should just go away.

The two sets of concepts put forward here, which are based on research by my colleagues and myself at the Brunel Institute of Organisation and Social Studies, suggest that there is a strong danger that two things which have already started to come out in the wash are: adequate basic patient care; and the future of the nursing profession. These are important issues, whoever you happen to be. I would like to put forward a definition of 'patient' and go on to consider the consequences for nursing as a profession. That will, alas, involve a bit more defining, to do with the nature of work, the existence of work levels, and the nature of what is called 'professional work'.

### The Meaning of 'Patient'

Recent work carried out here and in France* on the nature of domiciliary care and the conditions under which 'hospital' care can be provided at home[1] rapidly brought out the fact that we did not know nearly precisely enough just whom or what we were discussing.

---

*A grant from the Nuffield Foundation in connection with research in France is gratefully acknowledged.

147

Organisational talk is meaningless until the work to be done can be stated. It was therefore necessary to consider what being a patient really meant, and to follow that with some precision as to what a 'patient' needs.

What is a patient? To say it is someone who is sick is too easy. We know that probably the majority of people who feel themselves at some point to be ill do not go anywhere near a professional or a service.[2] They do not become patients: they remain ill people only.

The definition of 'patient' which I propose is: someone who feels he needs medical or related help; *and* who is accepted by a doctor as needing such help. If the doctor disagrees (nonsense, it's just tiredness/growing pains/'natural'), then the individual does not become a patient. If he does, however, what then?

## What are Patients' Needs?

Consequences begin to appear for the nursing world when we consider what being a patient involves. Is there any really general statement that can be made about this? Given that we confine ourselves to those with physical symptoms only (for it is in any case ever more doubtful whether psychological 'illness' is a correct view of those unsolved emotional problems which each of us copes with as best we can), I believe that being a physical patient will be found *always* to entail the following minimum:

(1) medical surveillance — by definition: if there is no medical surveillance then no patient exists;

(2) food — maybe ordinary, maybe special;

(3) physical comfort — adequate physical circumstances to be ill in, so far as furniture, warmth, etc. are concerned;

(4) human company — the presence of others to *some* degree; the normal person does not live totally apart from others even if living alone;

(5) nursing — basic looking after and basic nursing skills to keep the patient comfortable, attend to dressings and carry out simple procedures;

(6) 'emotional co-ordination of experience as patient' — the function of helping a patient to understand and cope with being ill, mainly dealt with by discussion with doctor(s) and nurses — or else this function is left to the patient, in which case he bears his anxieties alone. This may or may not be a problem for

any given person in any given state.

These six components need immediate comment: first, it can be seen
that items (2) (3) and (4) (food, physical comfort and human
contact) may be no more than anyone ordinarily needs, whether
a patient or not. In other words, these three constitute the package
we might call basic human needs in our particular society at this
point in history. It is striking that these particular items do not
figure prominently in any discussion of patients *in hospital*: there
they are taken for granted. They do not very much preoccupy staff,
patients or those who describe hospital work. But if a domiciliary
context for the treatment is proposed, it is precisely these basics which
first claim the attention of patient and family: how are these
needs to be met? Who will be there to attend to simple daily needs?

It is of fundamental importance that these basic human needs
should be recognised as forming *part of* being a patient – they are
not 'social needs', to be split off and assigned to other people and
other agencies: to the extent that they are dealt with in this way,
the person will feel split and dehumanised. As in the case of patients
admitted to hospital, such needs always appropriately *remain the
responsibility of health services* to meet for patients. Of course, it
does not invariably follow that all such needs have in practice to be
met by health service staff: obviously a large proportion of
patients can meet them by themselves. But the needs are there,
none the less. The only question is whether this person is a patient
or not. If yes, how are his basic patient needs being met?

I have said nothing about special patient needs – the needs for
diagnostic or treatment work which arise not because the patient is
a patient but because of his particular condition. We cannot pursue
these here, except to note that distinguishing basic and special
patient needs allows us to proceed to a further distinction: that
between 'full-time' and 'part-time' patients, which in turn makes it
possible to discuss the organisation of hospital and domiciliary
work on a basis which is independent of diagnosis.[3]

Where do nursing auxiliaries come in? There is a widespread feeling
that the work of auxiliaries is in some important sense different
from that of qualified nurses, but it remains hard to state exactly
what that difference is. A number of propositions are commonly
put forward to clarify the nature of the difference. For example,
it is sometimes said to be a matter of economies in service, of 'making
do' with less good staff, with less skilled work, with less training or

pay or status. I suggest that the problem is *not* fundamentally to do with any of them.

First, if we want work of specified kinds to be done for patients at a specified standard, then there are no alternatives. Any alternative is simply an acceptance of some other work or some other standard. Second, skill is not to be confused with the problem facing us here. Quite straightforward work can require great *skill,* which refers only to the precision, fineness or deftness of the work done, whatever its kind. Last, training, status, pay, uniform, titles — these follow from what we decide the work is to be: they cannot of themselves determine it.

If none of these factors assists us to pin down the difference between auxiliary nursing and professional nursing, what then is the problem? I propose that we are confronted here by a missing concept: the existence of *levels of work.* This is where the second group of definitions comes in.

They have to do with work and professionalisation. Basic nursing is increasingly different from the work that SRNs are trained for. Now the trend to regard basic nursing work as somehow no longer clearly part of the sphere of concern of the nursing profession is leading some nurses, doctors and the public to ask: if 'nursing' no longer includes the basic looking-after, if many of the important tasks which need to be done for the sick are called 'non-nursing duties' and assigned to less well-regarded groups of staff, what then is the basis of the 'nursing duties' which *are* part of the province of the nursing profession?

Our work is bringing to light the existence of an underlying basic structure in terms of which all employment work can be described.[4]

For our purposes it may be enough to remind you of the feeling of relief when someone tells you *exactly* what to do and how to do it (rapidly followed for some people by boredom and revolution if you have to go on following instructions too long), as against the more challenging but more demanding experience of being left to judge for yourself what to do and how to go about it and whether what you produce is any good or not. My colleagues have found a simple way of describing such experiences, and have found two things which are of consequence in this context: first, that there are very clear divisions between different levels of work; and second, that *professional* work seems to acquire that label only with work which is one level up from basic. Taken together, these findings

mean that the basic nursing touched on in the definition lies mainly
in the first level, while the more specialised 'professional' work
lies mainly in the second. It also needs to be said that human
capacity seems to match these levels, some of us at any given time
being at this level or that level (development does go on), and that,
whatever your level, you cannot in reality work at any other, up or
down.

Putting together the two sets of concepts, the following picture
begins to emerge. Both basic nursing and professional work are
called 'care'; 'nursing' is equally stretched across the same wide
spectrum of work levels, while SRNs, SENs and auxiliaries
probably concentrate in different sections of the field.

Figure 1

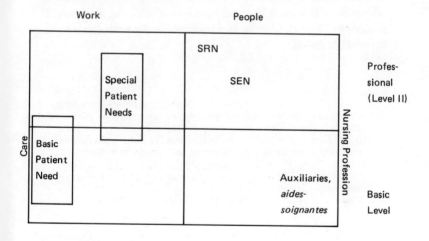

In some countries, the attempt is made to reserve the term 'nursing' to
the work of qualified nurses, leaving the 'basic-level' work to
non-nurses: this is true of Kenya and Portugal. But the awkward issue
which then arises for the nursing profession is this: if basic nursing
(basic-level work) is included as part of nursing, does that make its
claims to parity with other professions less strong? On the other
hand, if it cuts its ties with that level of work, does it not lose its
very title to consideration as a clear-cut field of activity, rooted in
that work of care of the sick which our concept of the patient

and his basic needs now re-emphasises?

One possibility is that a rapid separation is developing, whereby such factors as the changing status and opportunities for women, the opening up of new fields of work within the medical and related areas,[5] and not least the changing relative status of basic caring versus high technology are all contributing to create two groups. These would be a first group whose work is largely in the basic level, supervised by its senior members in the professional level, and a second group, whose aspirations and development would lead them away from such work, taking on managerial or developmental activities in the second or higher levels. Whether the single label 'nursing' will continue to be meaningfully attached to both such groups remains to be seen.

This is barely enough to raise the problems, let alone embark on a discussion of possible solutions. But perhaps enough has been said to show that there are tools in existence which at least make it possible to begin to describe and take hold of the problems we have just reviewed.

## Notes

1. Stephen Cang, 'Full-time and part-time patients: an analysis of patient needs and their implications for domiciliary and institutional care' in Brunel HSORU *Essays on Health Service Organisation* (London, Heinemann, forthcoming); Stephen Cang and Freda Clarke, *Hospital at Home* (London, Croom Helm, forthcoming); Stephen Cang and Freda Clarke, *Home Care of the Sick — an emerging general analysis based on schemes in France* (forthcoming).
2. G. Stimson and B. Webb: 'Going to See the Doctor' in *Medical Care*, Vol.3, No.1 (1965).
3. See Stephen Cang, op.cit.
4. Details can be found in the following publications: E. Jaques, *A General Theory of Bureaucracy* (London, Heinemann, 1976); R.W. Rowbottom and D. Billis, 'Stratification of Work and Organisational Design', *Human Relations*, Vol.30, No.1 (1977), pp.53-76; Brunel HSORU, *Essays on Health Service Organisation.*
5. Department of Health and Social Security, *The Extending Role of the Clinical Nurse*, Health Circular HC(77)22 (1977).

# 2 THE DEVELOPMENT OF A PLAN FOR NURSING CARE IN RESIDENTIAL HOMES

## Margaret Irvine (Northern Ireland)

The area of the Northern Health and Social Services Board comprises the areas of the former local authorities of County Londonderry, County Antrim (excluding Lisburn Borough) and part of Belfast. The population is 340,000, with a preponderance of the younger age groups. There are both urban and rural communities, industrial and agricultural, radical and conservative, 'troubled' and 'less troubled' by civil unrest.

The social services' inheritance from the Board was excellent in regard to number of places for residents and the present Development Plan (1976) will allow replacement of existing sub-standard accommodation. The increasing frailty of the residents was, however, a problem for the authorities in regard to the allocation of appropriate staff and resources. This was confirmed by the dependency survey which was carried out as part of the work of the Strategic Planning Team, with consulting assistance from Dr Barr, Oxford Regional Board, which preceded the Development Plan.[1] Tables 1, 2 and 3 summarise their findings.

The question, 'Are beds used properly?' revealed that hospital beds were being taken up by patients who strictly did not require hospital care. It was inferred that this care was a substitute for more appropriate community care. High admission rates in some localities may be attributed partly to the fact that beds were available locally.

### Consideration of the Problems

A special sub-committee was set up at the Northern Ireland Department to examine nurse/patient staffing ratios and nursing manpower. The role and function of the nursing auxiliary/ward assistant was considered and a tabulation of suggested duties for these grades was drawn up and passed to the Central Committee for consideration.

At the same time the role of the nurse in residential homes was being examined, and a Northern Ireland Residential Social Work Liaison Group was formed in the spring of 1975. Its membership comprised: representatives of the Association of Social Workers, the Residential Care Association, the Royal College of Nursing and the staff of training schools in the province. They collated and analysed information relating to: number of statutory facilities, number of non-statutory facilities, numbers and categories of residents, staff and their education, and voluntary workers.

The characteristics of the residents in the homes for the elderly were examined in the social work framework. This examination resulted in a census of all residents modelled on that used by Carstairs and Morrison (Scottish Health Services Study, No.19) for their report, *The Elderly in Residential Care.* The findings confirmed those of the previously mentioned dependency study.

## Groundwork for Problem-solving

### (a) Development of Hospital Services Plan

As a result of the decision to concentrate acute hospital services at two points (Antrim and Coleraine), there emerged a need for a supporting hospital in each local population.

### (b) Residential Staff Census

This revealed a preponderance of nursing qualifications at senior level, whilst at caring and assistant caring staff levels, there were practically no qualifications of any description recorded. No member of staff in either the statutory or non-statutory homes had a relevant full-time social work qualification. Only six staff were recorded as having attended the In-service Study Scheme out of a total of 825 residential social workers in post.

These facts demonstrate the traditional high level of importance which is given to the physical care of the elderly and physically handicapped resident and the importance of nursing input into this type of home. In policy terms, however, this finding raises important issues as to the objectives of these establishments, of how the needs of residents are perceived, and of how the residential tasks are defined and carried out. Are residential homes for the elderly and physically handicapped extensions of the geriatric hospital service or units of 'alternative living' for those who can no longer be supported in the community?

It is significant that in the recent survey conducted in preparation for *The Report on the Development of Hospital Services in the Area for the Northern Health and Social Services Board,* it was recorded that 'of 712 residents. . .34 residents (4.8 per cent) were considered to require care more appropriate to hospital.' In the light of these facts it would seem that a review of the objectives, staffing and training for the staff in homes for the elderly and physically handicapped is called for.

### (c) Census of Residents

A majority of residents were found to be able to undertake self-care activities — washing, dressing, toileting and feeding. A majority could feed themselves, three-quarters could toilet themselves and almost three-quarters could wash themselves. Dressing presented the most difficulty. Men were more able generally than women. Overall, 37 per cent of men and 23 per cent of women were considered capable of managing their own medications. Severe mental confusion, which would probably preclude self-care and self-management capabilities, was assessed at a level of 6.9 per cent of men and 14 per cent of women.

The recommendation for a periodic repeat census of residents (to include private and voluntary homes) is made as a result of the social work analysis. This would attempt to ensure that planning could keep pace with change in the conditions, and therefore the needs, of the frail elderly.[2]

### Outcomes to Date

(1) The Development of Hospital Services Plan has been accepted and the need to look at nurse training has been made a priority.

(2) Social Services have redrafted the staffing structure for care attendants, including senior care attendants. The prime responsibility of the care attendant will be the personal care of residents. This includes bathing, washing, shaving, washing hair, dressing, toileting, feeding residents who require such assistance. These are duties similar to those of ward orderlies in hospital wards for the elderly, and were delineated as a result of ward activity sampling.

(3) A working party has been set up to prepare a training course leading to the Certificate in Social Service.

### The Recognition of Key Questions

Basically the ideas of experts in different disciplines were the same, and the following were recommended:

a career structure for care attendants;
care teams allocated to small groups of residents;
training which would avoid 'the nursing model' for residential care
staff.

However, in any movement towards the above recommendations, there
are key questions to be answered. Can social and nursing care be
differentiated, and on what basis? How can the nursing care required in
residential accommodation be identified, quantified and provided? How
feasible is dividing labour and specialisation of function within the size
of team required in a 50- or 60-place unit? Must further consideration be
given to the problem of optimum size for living accommodation? To what
extent should health care involvement affect the management of
residential accommodation as social units? How best to preserve the
rights of individuals to receive and refuse — to choose — care? To what
extent should the social services expand into responsibilities for the frail
elderly, especially the confused elderly?

In consideration of these critical questions, and within the
implementation process of the Development Plan, it is hoped that the
call for continued research will not be a vain one.

## Notes

1. Northern Health and Social Services Board, *Development of Services in the
   Area of the Northern Health and Social Services Board*, report of the
   Strategic Planning Team, Ballymena, Northern Ireland (1976).
2. Social Work Advisory Group for the DHSS, Northern Ireland, *The Need for
   Care: Personal Social Services in Northern Ireland* (1977).

### Table 1: Analysis of Hospital Surveys

| Specialty | Total Patients in Survey | Did not require Hospital Care | | Required Hospital Care | | Required Hospital Care Technical | | Mainly Nursing | |
|---|---|---|---|---|---|---|---|---|---|
| | | No. | Per Cent | No. | Per Cent | No. | Per Cent | No. | Per Cer |
| Medicine | 638 | 82 | 13 | 556 | 87 | 398 | 72 | 158 | 28 |
| Surgery | 606 | 35 | 6 | 571 | 94 | 465 | 81 | 106 | 19 |
| ENT | 48 | 2 | 4 | 46 | 96 | 46 | 100 | — | — |
| Gynaecology | 113 | 7 | 6 | 106 | 94 | 102 | 96 | 4 | 4 |
| GP and Geriatrics | 1,392 | 344 | 25 | 1,048 | 75 | 20 | 2 | 1,028 | 98 |
| Total | 2,797 | 470 | 17 | 2,327 | 83 | 1,031 | 44 | 1,296 | 56 |

The Social Services Residences Survey covered a total of 712 residents and the results are shown in Table 2. Thirty-four residents (4.8 per cent) were considered to require care more appropriate to hospital, although they were being provided in the residences with the necessary level of care. In practice, the criteria for transfer from Social Services residences to hospital were higher than those adopted for direct admission to or for retention in hospital. A shortage of staff or other factors might, however, lead to a need for hospital accommodation for some 5 per cent of residents.

Source: All tables from *Development of Hospital Services in the Area of the Northern Health and Social Services Board* (1976), pp.88-9.

## Table 2: Analysis of Survey in Social Services Residential Facilities

| Total Residents in Survey | | Residents Potentially Requiring Hospital In-Patient Care | |
|---|---|---|---|
| No. | Per Cent | No. | Per Cent |
| 712 | 100 | 34 | 4.8 |

The survey of patients at home covered a total of 2,696 patients visited by District Nurses and the results are shown in Table 3. The care given by families and District Nurses resulted in 129 (4.9 per cent) patients being kept at home when they might reasonably have been in hospital. A breakdown of family health or other change in circumstances might lead to a transfer to hospital.

## Table 3: Analysis of Survey for Patients at Home

| Total Patients in Survey | | Patients Potentially Requiring Hospital In-Patient Care | |
|---|---|---|---|
| No. | Per Cent | No. | Per Cent |
| 2,696 | 100 | 129 | 4.9 |

Summary. Both admissions and out-patient attendances at hospitals increased between 1964 and 1973. The work-load of the supporting services correspondingly increased. The rise in the number of admissions was accommodated by an increase in beds, and some reduction in length of stay, but generally by an increased throughput. Occupancy in many specialties remained lower than optimum. Only in geriatrics did the admissions decrease, because the increase in bed numbers could not compensate for the longer length of stay. Five per cent of the elderly sick at home and in Social Services residences were potential hospital patients. The slow throughput of geriatric beds had an effect on the number of long-stay patients in the acute beds in general hospitals.

A substantial number of patients went to Belfast hospitals, not only for Regional Services, but also for services which would normally be provided locally. The numbers admitted to the Royal Belfast Hospital for Sick Children reflects the lack of established paediatric services in the Northern Board Area.

The local catchments of hospitals corresponded to the scattered distribution of the present hospital pattern. The volume and direction of patient flows will be taken into account in our recommendations for any new hospital pattern.

Dependency studies to show the use of beds indicated that hospital beds were being taken up by patients who strictly did not require hospital care and it is inferred that this care was a substitute for more appropriate community care. High admission rates in some localities may be attributed partly to the fact that beds were available locally.

# 3 THE ROLE OF THE NURSING AUXILIARY — A CASE FOR RESTRICTION

Morag Lambert (Scotland)

In recent years statistics have shown a great increase in the number of 'other nurses' employed within the National Health Service — in Scotland in all general hospitals the total number of nursing auxiliaries in 1970 was 6,360[1] (whole-time equivalents) and in 1975, 10,868[2] (WTE). According to Brian Watkin,[3] one in four of all personnel giving nursing care in hospitals and the community are untrained nursing auxiliary/assistant staff. Increasing also are the criticisms of the standards of nursing care which patients are receiving in hospitals. These two facts lead to the title of this paper. I consider this restriction in terms of three aspects:

(1) the restriction in the number of nursing auxiliary staff employed in the NHS;
(2) the restriction of the job of the nursing auxiliary;
(3) the restriction in the title nursing auxiliary.

Limitation of the number of nursing auxiliaries is surely an essential, if the standards of patient care are to improve and be of a high quality. This is not meant as a disparagement to those auxiliaries who are caring for people and who in many instances give invaluable help in the hospital wards, clinics, and in the care of patients in the community. Tables 1 and 2 show the number of nursing auxiliaries employed in three areas of Scotland in 1975. I have shown the number of qualified staff against the number of nursing auxiliary staff and have purposely excluded nurses in training. This is because the qualified staff and auxiliary staff are the permanent members of the ward team, while the nurses-in-training are fluctuating members of staff.

Nursing care should be of a higher standard if given by a qualified nurse or nurse in training, rather than an unqualified, untrained member of staff. If not, why train nurses? It must also be obvious that if the ratio of other nurses to qualified nurses is high, the care given to patients must be of a lesser standard than we would wish and nursing auxiliaries, who in many instances have received no form of training at all, are put in the position of carrying out duties quite outwith their

Table 1: General Hospitals (whole-time equivalents)

| Area | Qualified Staff | Auxiliary Staff | Percentage Qualified Staff/Nursing Auxiliaries |
|---|---|---|---|
| GGHB | 2,926 | 3,247 | 47 : 53 |
| Lothian Health Board | 1,950 | 1,612 | 54 : 46 |
| Highland Health Board | 450 | 339 | 57 : 43 |

Table 2: Mental Hospitals (whole-time equivalents)

| Area | Qualified Staff | Auxiliary Staff | Percentage Qualified Staff/Nursing Auxiliaries |
|---|---|---|---|
| GGHB | 841 | 684 | 55 : 45 |
| Lothian Health Board | 563 | 496 | 53 : 47 |
| Highland Health Board | 190 | 128 | 60 : 40 |

These tables show a fairly similar pattern of employment of these grades of staff throughout the country.

scope and capabilities. This must be to the detriment of patient care and also to the detriment of the morale of qualified nurses, who realise the dangers inherent in the situation. At a time when qualified nursing staff may be experiencing some difficulty in finding the employment of their choice, especially married staff who are not as mobile as the unmarried and who also are increasing in number, it is an opportune moment for restricting the number of auxiliary nurses employed within the National Health Service. This could be achieved either by eliminating them through non-replacement, or by assimilation into nurse training.

The job the nursing auxiliary does should be clearly defined. This may be difficult, as there are many essential procedures which are carried out by all grades of staff, but it is vital that their responsibility to the patient is clearly delineated and their role and work clearly outlined. Whatever they do, it is important that they are given instructions, whether it is the practical aspect of the job, how to communicate with people, or how to care for the sick. Also, some reasoning behind these instructions must be given, so that they fully understand what to do and so that the duties they carry out are done as they ought to be done. We must give them the opportunity to practise what is taught. We must ensure that before becoming permanent members of the establishment we are certain that they have the necessary degree of responsibility for the job they are employed to do. In no way do I see a term of training lasting several months with certification at the end of it. If they have the intelligence and capabilities to achieve this then they should be encouraged to train for a statutory nursing qualification. In the past we have been negligent in the teaching of this grade of staff and this is surely an indictment of our profession. What other profession employs large groups of untrained personnel to carry out the work of that same profession?

The title nursing auxiliary should be reconsidered — we never address this member of staff as nursing auxiliary — we very often call her 'Nurse' — a title she has no legal right to, as indicated in the Nurses (Scotland) Act 1951 and the Nurses Act 1957, which states:

> Any person who, not being a duly registered nurse or a duly enrolled nurse, takes or uses the name or title of nurse, either alone or in combination with any other words or letters, shall be liable on summary conviction to a fine. . .[4]

It is an anomaly if someone with no professional standing can use this title. The name should only be used when a statutory qualification has been gained. We should jealously guard the right to the use of this title, especially when we have trained and worked hard over a lengthy period of time to gain the right to call ourselves nurses.

Restriction of this group of staff must surely enhance our profession, for at present the nursing auxiliaries represent 35 per cent of the established work-force in the general field. Could we not reduce

Table 3: Scotland 1975 (whole-time equivalents)

| Qualified Staff | Nurses in Training | Nursing Auxiliaries |
|---|---|---|
| 11,688 | 7.938 | 10.868 |
| 38.33 per cent | 26.03 per cent | 35.64 per cent |

Source: Scottish Home and Health Department, *Scottish Health Statistics, 1975.*

this figure to a maximum of 20 per cent of the nursing work-force? Numbers could be limited by either assimilating into our training schools the auxiliaries of the necessary calibre (and the introduction of

ie Briggs recommendations for an initial 18-month training for the
ertificate of Nursing Practice would simplify this) or, by natural
astage, reduce the numbers considerably. How can we be members of a
ring profession and be so uncaring in the use of so many untrained
embers of staff? Apart from giving them the title nurse and using
em in large numbers, we also give them, in some instances,
sponsibilities quite beyond their remit or capabilities. This is
amaging not only to patient care but maybe to their own personal
:alth and job satisfaction.

Let us carefully consider a case for restriction of these 'other' nurses,
hich would be of benefit to the nursing profession and – of prime
aportance – of benefit to the patient.

**otes**

Scottish Home and Health Department, *Scottish Health Statistics, 1970.*
Scottish Home and Health Department, *Scottish Health Statistics, 1975.*
B. Watkins, in *Nursing Mirror,* 30 June 1977.
Nurses (Scotland) Act, 1951; Nurses Act, 1957.

# 4 THE ROLE OF THE NURSING AUXILIARIES IN THE CARING TEAM

## Norman Martin (England)

In the United Kingdom, the term 'nursing auxiliary' refers to employment in the general nursing field and 'nursing assistant' to employment in the psychiatric field. For this paper, nursing auxiliary will be used to designate workers in both environments. The feminine gender has been used to refer to the auxiliary, though both males and females are so employed.

Briefly, the main point in the official definition is that a nursing auxiliary is an unqualified person who is engaged in nursing duties under the supervision of a qualified nurse and who is not a student or a pupil nurse. This description must, of course, be opened out to produce the practical role this grade of staff are engaged in.

There are no national criteria for selection of nursing auxiliaries, so that they form an extremely diverse group of people. Couple this with the various work situations and the equally various ideas of management as to the most effective way in which the auxiliary may be utilised in the wards or departments, and we have the basic problems in defining the role of auxiliaries.

The position a nursing auxiliary holds in some quarters is in doubt. Has she anything to do with nursing, or is she merely a go-between, to be used as and when or where needed, regardless of the job? This is a matter of concern and must at all costs be put in the right perspective. The position of an auxiliary should be in no doubt. She must be part of the caring team. Even if it is at the bottom rung of the ladder – someone must be at the bottom. First-year learners are at the start of their career but they will proceed, one hopes upwards. The auxiliary remains a stable and in many cases a long-term member of the team. It is only fair to say that the majority of auxiliaries realise the limitations of their position and also the very diverse situations in which they find themselves. They appear to be a thin wedge lodged between the domestic at the lower end and learners at the higher end.

In that the nursing auxiliary is recognised as a member of the caring team, her function is to assist and give support to the nurses within the team as required. If everyone in the caring team has been trained to co-ordinate their efforts to achieve a common objective, the auxiliary's contribution of many items of basic care, though not demanding great skill, is essential to the patient. This affords the qualified staff greater opportunity to use their skills and expertise towards ultimate improvement in patient care.

The balance of staff in the team obviously depends upon the work situation. In acute areas, where a high level of dependency exists, nursing auxiliaries may be nil, rising to 30 per cent as a reasonable balance in areas such as geriatric nursing. We all know of the situation in which the percentage is nearer eighty. This indicates that each work situation must be assessed at local level.

The question is, 'Are nursing auxiliaries required?' The answer can be found as we assess the increasing demands made on the nursing profession by the technical knowledge and passing down of medical procedures. The present-day professional is moving further and further away from the basic bedside care of the sick, such as attending to the feeding of patients, toilet, or comfort in and out of bed.

As it is generally agreed that auxiliaries are required to assist with basic nursing care of patients in many spheres of work, the most effective form of training will be that given on or near the job, training provided by and within the organisation. As the specific needs of trainees will vary considerably, a pre-service training programme will have to be planned to cover those aspects of their work which are common to all. Further training designed to meet the special needs of staff according to their place of work will also have to be designed. Training in the work situation is vital for certain specific skills and avoids the problems associated with the transference of learning often encountered by this grade of staff. This means, too, that the initial pre-service training can be of a very general nature. As an association we have for some time recommended an ideal additional training which provides a wider coverage of relevant subjects. These are the courses in home nursing, initial and advanced, of the British Red Cross Society.

The overall aims of any syllabus produced are recommended as follows:

(1) to enable the new auxiliary to appreciate the scope and importance of her work as an essential part of the total service given to the patient;

(2) to introduce the auxiliary to her duties and to enable her to develop skill in simple basic nursing techniques;

(3) to warn the auxiliary of the possible consequences of undertaking

tasks outside her sphere of responsibility.

Local circumstances must be taken into account and the particular
training and experience of individuals may affect the amount of
responsibility which they can be given.
   Job descriptions, bearing in mind what has been mentioned so
far, could be made up from the following heads:

   the patient at home and in hospital;
   the hospital and its departments;
   the patient's surroundings;
   the patient's comfort;
   exercise and rest;
   the patient's excretions;
   food and fluids;
   first aid;
   emergency procedures;
   the care of the dying;
   extra for maternity areas     — baby care
                                 — labour and delivery rooms;
   extra for psychiatric areas   — Mental Health Act
                                   mental disorders
                                   participation in the patient's day.


It can be seen, surely, that nursing auxiliaries should be trained to a
certain level. They are not asking for or expecting to be a third tier
of nursing, just to be trained to do the job of a nursing auxiliary.
   A nursing auxiliary should always be under the supervision of a
qualified nurse, but this presents difficulties similar to those to do with
training, as supervision must also relate to the problems of staff
balance. The ideal situation, and one in which it is possible to find a
working solution, is to assume the ratio is one-third auxiliaries,
the remainder being students, pupils and qualified. The qualified,
of course, are registered and enrolled. A qualified nurse need not be
far away even if the auxiliary is assisting a student nurse. The
question is, how far away can the supervision be? How often and
how constant or at frequent or infrequent rounds? We are back to the
situation of local need, the type of work area and the auxiliary
herself. Under no circumstances should an auxiliary be left
alone on a ward 'in charge', regardless of the area of work.
The immediate response to this is to ask about the auxiliary working

in the community. Here the position is treated in a different way. The Nursing Officer would deploy her auxiliaries to patients who require the care an auxiliary could give. The patient would be seen by a qualified nurse to assess the need and instruction given to the auxiliary on a daily report basis. Frequent visits to the patient by a qualified nurse would be made to ensure the auxiliary was working within her training and capabilities. In fact, the auxiliary fits in well in the community field, relieving the qualified nurse to care for the patient requiring a higher content of nursing.

Nursing auxiliaries have been with us for a very long time. Under a variety of names, no doubt, but with us just the same. Many people look upon the auxiliary as a new grade having just crept in the back door. The present-day auxiliary has a definite role to play in caring for the sick. They have been there all along doing just that, but they need to be organised and integrated into the caring team.

# 5 AUXILIARY NURSING PERSONNEL IN PORTUGAL: EVOLUTION OF THE SITUATION AND TRENDS

Maria Teresa Quintão Pereira Barreira Antunes
Maria Arlete Teixeira de Sousa
Mariana Dulce Diníz de Sousa

## 1. Introduction

We shall present here a brief summary of the setting up of auxiliary nurse courses, the evolution of this professional category, and its role within Portuguese nursing. It will focus, also, on the demands made by this nursing personnel, the role played by the unions, the abolition of this category and the setting up of the courses for promotion of auxiliary nurses to nurses.

It seems relevant to present a brief explanatory note about auxiliary nursing personnel in Portugal. In this country, in addition to Category I nurses, as defined by the ICN, there are auxiliary nurses, Category II (ICN), whose training is equivalent to the British SEN, and a third category of other auxiliary nursing personnel. The latter group, nursing aides and public health aides, may be considered Category III (ICN), but are not considered nursing personnel in Portugal.

## 2. Auxiliary Nurse Courses

Until 1947 nursing care in Portugal was mainly carried out by nurses, after a two-year training following four years' schooling. In 1947 both entrance requirements were increased to six years' schooling and length of training was increased to three years. At this time training for auxiliary nurses, of one year's duration, was started in order to compensate for the shortage of nurses and to relieve them of those tasks of a less responsible nature. In 1952 that training was increased to eighteen months, as after the first twelve months, a six-month period of practical experience was required.

In 1965 the reform of nursing education altered the structure of training for auxiliary nurses. Entrance requirements were increased to six years' schooling and at the same time entrance requirements for nurse training were increased to nine years' schooling.

The structure of auxiliary nurse training was aimed at preparing this personnel to give general nursing care (hygiene, comfort and attending to basic needs) and to give some special nursing care of a less responsible nature.

Auxiliary nurse training was always the responsibility of schools of nursing and, since 1965, these schools of nursing have been under the supervision and co-ordination of a central department responsible to the Secretary of State for Health.

### 3. Role Played by Auxiliary Nurses in Portuguese Nursing

In 1974, after the 25th April 'Revolution', the government decided to abolish auxiliary nurse training, following nation-wide demands made by this personnel. At this time, the number of auxiliary nurses was approximately double that of nurses.

Throughout the years few candidates sought nurse training. In an attempt to solve the problem of nursing staff shortage, the government promoted the training of less qualified and cheaper personnel, not only in terms of training but also in terms of salaries. Several schools of nursing were opened which carried out auxiliary nurse training exclusively.

Several other interlinked aspects about the situation of Portuguese nursing should be mentioned. A lack of proper definition of functions both of health workers, and especially of nursing personnel, led to nurses practising some aspects of medicine, nursing functions being carried out by auxiliary nurses, and the taking over of nursing care by untrained personnel. Auxiliary nurse training was carried out in a much greater depth than that expected and desirable for this type of course by some schools of nursing. It was argued by the auxiliary nurses that there was a need to prepare them for the reality of life, as they contended that they were required to carry out nursing care of great responsibility.

Nurses occupied mainly leadership posts, i..e. staff nurse upwards. (It must be remembered that student nurses in Portugal have student status and consequently health services are staffed only by trained personnel.) They carried out mainly administrative tasks, leaving direct nursing care to auxiliary nurses. The latter were mainly given the less desirable shifts, evening and night, as nurses kept the morning shifts to themselves. The usual shifts for many years have been 8 a.m.–4 p.m.; 4 p.m. – 12 midnight; 12 midnight – 8 a.m. It can be said that for many years hardly a nurse could be found on duty after 4 p.m. in any hospital throughout Portugal.

It is true to affirm that auxiliary nurses, initially intended to carry out nursing care of a less responsible nature under the supervision of nurses, were increasingly found to be playing the role of nurse.

## 4. The Auxiliary Nurses' 'Movement'

It is difficult to determine the exact time when the auxiliary nurses initiated their 'movement' aimed at their own promotion to the status of nurse. However, in 1968 these auxiliaries organised a nation-wide movement leading to the presentation to the government of a document stating their situation and making great demands. The government ignored these demands and the auxiliary nurses decided to further press the government by using such measures as refusing to carry out those nursing tasks which should be carried out by nurses. Their demands were greatly supported by the medical profession who, at the time, were also pressing the government with requests of their own.

In September 1971, in an attempt to meet the demands made by auxiliary nursing personnel, the government passed legislation structuring nursing careers which allowed the auxiliary nurses to become nurses, provided they passed a special course.

It was not until August 1972 that this course was established — Course for Promotion of Auxiliary Nurses to Nurses. It is of twenty months' duration, full-time and administered by Schools of Nursing. The first intake of students was the following October but only a very small number of students were admitted. This was due not only to difficulties of Schools of Nursing, in terms of size, but also to the fact that health services could not release a greater number of auxiliary nurses.

The auxiliary nurses were not happy with this state of affairs, as it would take years before all the auxiliary nurses could attend the course. This was made worse by the fact that the auxiliary nurse course was still being taught. The April 'Revolution' in 1974 offered this personnel group new opportunities to press their claims. Many of these people wished to become nurses 'overnight', while many others wished a shorter period of further training to be made available to greater numbers of auxiliary nurses. These could be carried out in multiple centres and afford the possibility of combining work and study. At the same time the nursing unions, ineffective until April 1974, found conditions appropriate to support the great majority of their members, the auxiliary nurses, in their claims. The unions put forward a new promotion course which started in February 1975.

The abolition of the auxiliary nurse course led to the abolition of this same category. The auxiliary nurses who were considered by the unions as having carried out nurses' functions for three years became 'third grade' nurses, after which they were allowed to attend the promotion course.

## 5. Course for Promotion of 'Third Grade' Nurses (Ex-auxiliary Nurses)

This course, which started in 1975, is of an essentially theoretical nature, containing those practical aspects considered necessary by the people who attend it. This course lasts eight months with an average of three hours of educational activities daily, co-ordinated with working hours.

A national committee was set up, its terms of reference being to study needs and resources for administration of the course in order to set up training centres all over the country. Its terms of reference included also the supervision, co-ordination and evaluation of these training centres which can operate within Schools of Nursing, Hospitals or Health Centres which are accredited by the National Committee.

This promotion course confers the title of nurse, allowing the people who complete it to proceed in this career. It is expected that the course will cease to operate in 1980 when every auxiliary nurse should have had the opportunity to complete it.

## 6. Other Auxiliary Nursing Personnel

Portugal has deployed other auxiliary nursing personnel under the supervision of nursing personnel. In hospitals these personnel are called nursing aides and in community services are called public health aides.

The nursing aides followed a four-month practical in-service training aimed at preparing them to help the nurses by carrying out simple tasks which do not involve specific nursing knowledge, such as those relating to hygiene, comfort, care of material and equipment and environmental safety. The public health aides also followed a four-month training in community services aimed at preparing them to work in health centres which are concerned mainly with primary care.

Although this type of personnel were to perform only auxiliary tasks under the supervision of nurses, the lack of well-organised teams and lack of qualified nurses has led to the performance of nursing tasks by this same personnel. It is obvious that this fact could lead to demands by this personnel wishing to be admitted into the career structure. However, this has not been allowed. These personnel were encouraged to do nurse training provided they fulfilled entrance requirements. In the meantime the preparation of this personnel has completely stopped.

This country's experience concerning the use of auxiliary nurses permits us to argue that it is unwise to organise specific programmes or courses for this personnel group; they should only be given in-service training. However, this group should be auxiliary to health personnel generally, and not only to nurses.

It can be concluded that Portugal has chosen to have one-level nursing personnel only, similar to medicine and the other health professions.

# 6 CARING AND SHARING: THE JOINT USE OF TRAINING AND MANPOWER RESOURCES BETWEEN SOCIAL SERVICE AND HEALTH SERVICE

M.E.F. Perkins (England)

The title of this paper is simple enough. This caring and sharing as human beings we are doing every day of our lives. As people, the one thing we are certain of, from the taking of our first breath, is death, and even this encompasses many uncertainties: place, time, with whom, and from what cause. It is known that with care life may be preserved, prolonged and enhanced. We have experience of care: parental care, medical care, nursing care and self-care. Nevertheless, the job definition of a nurse is one of the most difficult to compose. Each of us present will have our own image of the nurse.

The nurse, like other professions, must have support staff. This is to enable the nurse to use his/her expertise to the greatest advantage — giving the benefit of her skill to the majority rather than the minority of people requiring care. The nursing auxiliary, aide, assistant or attendant is one person to whom the nurse looks for this support, as a means of extending her effect.

We are familiar with job descriptions. It appears that the job description of the nursing auxiliary is achieved by analysing the functional role of the nurse. Difficulties therefore arise if there is no generally acceptable job definition of the nurse. Hence the well-known expression 'non-nursing duties', evolved from the practice of subtracting all duties not pertaining to the technical role of the nurse from a holistic baseline. Paradoxically, this makes the nurse appear not to care for the person as a whole, despite the well-known phrase so often quoted by nurses about their role.

The word nursing in 'nursing auxiliary' could purposely be put into brackets. Is it necessary that a person who helps a nurse use the word nursing in his/her title? Is it not better to head your own level rather than to tail on at the end of another profession? This is especially relevant as the Joint Care Planning circular (HC(76)18/LAC(76)6) develops in practice.

171

## Social Services and Joint Care Planning

Home care workers/residential care workers/home helps are among the other titles found in the social services field. Joint care planning is largely involving and bringing together the general care and social services needs of a person living in the community. This may be in his or her own home or one of the special homes run by the special services department. Joint care planning requires new thinking, a new approach. In marrying two bodies together and preparing its workers, is it not the the right time to reconsider the multiplicity of titles, devising perhaps one title and one training?

## Proposed Outline of Training

A training scheme should be established in each area health authority for the training of 'residential care workers'. The effectiveness of the training would be monitored and reported to the joint care planning teams. The training syllabus would include:

(a)    procedures which can be carried out by care staff *with* the supervision of a qualified nurse;
(b)    procedures which can be carried out *without* the supervision of a qualified nurse.

The qualified nurse in a social services residential home could and, perhaps, should be a Level II (state enrolled nurse). This would relieve the first-level nurse (state registered nurse) to use her skills in the more acute care situation. A suggested framework of training could be: one week in a nurse education centre, one week community experience, one week in hospital night duty, and one week in residential accommodation.This then would be a joint care planning centre; salaries would be paid by social services and there would be use of health service facilities whilst training. Clothing would be as worn by social services workers, and the health service receive the services of community and hospital workers.

This can only result in:

(a)    better standard of care through training;
(b)    more efficient use of manpower resources;
(c)    preventing duplication of work;
(d)    better use of joint funding monies.

It is only experience through trial and error that will decide the role of both the nurse and the auxiliary in this new setting.

# 7 ONE ASPECT OF THE EMERGENCE AND GROWTH OF NURSING AUXILIARY EMPLOYMENT

B.L.E.C. Reedy (England)

My purpose is to present some data which may illuminate obliquely the emergence and role of the nursing auxiliary. The data relate only to qualified nurses working in the community in England and do not concern hospital nurses.

In Britain, community or 'district' nurses have traditionally worked mainly in patients' homes and since the early 1960s this has been increasingly in collaboration with general practitioners (GPs) and other members of the so-called 'primary care team'. Although small in number compared with the hospital nurses, the community nurses are relatively influential and have their own distinctive history and traditions. Since the National Health Service (NHS) began they have been employed by the local (now 'area') health authorities and, together with the community midwives and health visitors, have seen the provision of care in the patients' own homes as their principal commitment. In the past it was usual for district nurses and general practitioners to work almost independently of each other but during the last twenty years an arrangement has developed between the health authorities and the GPs whereby the nurses become 'attached' to a specified general practice and (in theory) responsible only for the patients of that practice. It was assumed that this would lead to a closer relationship between nurses and GPs as the basis for developing the primary health care team in the community.

For a number of reasons this hope has not yet been fully realised but as the result of a complete enumeration by postal questionnaire of the general practices in England in 1974[1] we have been able to show how the 'attachment' of community nurses to these practices has progressed since 1960 (Figure 1, interrupted line). At the time of the survey, 68 per cent of all the practices in England had one or more attached nurses (this does not include health visitors or midwives) although this proportion varied greatly between the ninety area health authorities (AHAs).

The position is complicated because GPs can also employ nurses themselves, independently of the health authorities, and be reimbursed

173

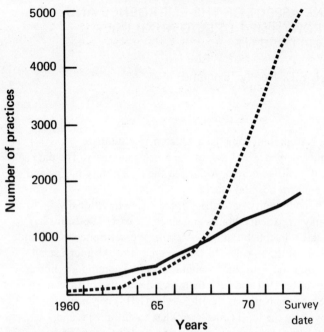

Figure 1: Nurses in General Practices in England, 1974

Number of practices starting attachment (-----) or employment (——) of nurses in each year.

Source: B.L.E.C. Reedy, P.R. Philips and P.J. Newell, 'Nurses and Nursing in Primary Medical Care in England', *British Medical Journal*, 2, (1976), pp.1304-6.

by the NHS to the extent of 70 per cent of the nurses' salaries. These are the so-called 'practice' nurses and Figure 1 (continuous line) shows that whilst 'attachment' was progressing, so also was an increase in the number of practices employing nurses. At the time of our survey, 3,100 nurses were employed by 24 per cent of the practices in England and these nurses numbered one-fifth of all the nurses working in the community at that time.

Our survey showed that the two kinds of nurse were *more* (not less) likely to coexist in the same practice and the descriptive literature suggests that they are responsible for complementary functions in the practices in which they both work. It is probable that the nurses employed by GPs work almost entirely in the treatment rooms of health centres and other practice premises and that they are particularly concerned with technical or hospital-orientated activities in which they could be said to be acting as assistants to the doctor whilst still appearing to retain their identity and status as nurses. Attached (health authority) nurses, on the other hand, have appeared to be mainly responsible for the home nursing element of the system with the accent on bedside nursing and care, although some were rumoured to take part in treatment room activities as well.

Recently we interviewed random samples of 'attached' and 'employed' nurses in nine area health authorities in England[2] and compared their activities. In Table 1 we have selected thirteen activities to show the proportions of each kind of nurse who had carried out each of these activities at least once during the month before the survey. The order of the activities is ranked from top to bottom of the table by the relative frequency with which the 'attached' nurses carried them out. This rank order can also be seen to coincide with a progressive change from 'caring' activities, traditionally the prerogative of nurses, to 'medical' activities, traditionally the prerogative of physicians. Furthermore, the activities at the top of the table can virtually only be carried out in patients' homes and the skills needed for them are taught during basic nurse training. The activities further down the list become increasingly difficult and inappropriate in the home because they need special equipment and some require emergency treatment to be available — as with the giving of desensitising injections. Nurses need special training after qualification for most of these activities. Finally, a comparison of the 'attached' and 'employed' nurses shows the anticipated predominance of the former in caring and of the latter in medical activities, but it is clear that the 'attached' nurses in our sample also had a recognisable commitment to these medical activities.

Table 2 analyses the changes in the number and location of the first (i.e. 'new') treatments given by community nurses employed by area health authorities in England during the period 1972 to 1975.[3,4] The sample of nurses on which the figures are based is not quite the same as that used in our own survey because it excluded treatments given by the nurses employed by GPs and not all of the nurses included were 'attached' to general practices. Nevertheless the data show a trend which is consistent between the years 1972 and 1975, although the intervening years have been omitted from the table. The figures relate only to qualified nurses and do not include the work of aides and auxiliaries.

Although the total number of new treatments has increased by 31 per cent over three years, the increase has been predominantly in health centres and other GP premises. Whereas a majority of first treatments were carried out in patients' homes in 1972, the position is reversed in 1975 and the rate of change was greatest in the health

Table 1: Activities of a Sample of Nurses During a Typical Month

|  | Proportion of Nurses Performing Each Activity | |
|---|---|---|
|  | Attached Nurses (per cent) | Employed Nurses (per cent) |
| Bathing | 95 | 0 |
| Assisting to lavatory, etc. | 91 | 7 |
| Treating bowel by enema/suppository | 91 | 10 |
| Catheterising | 59 | 6 |
| Feeding by hand | 40 | 0 |
| Syringing ears | 39 | 82 |
| Weighing patients | 37 | 81 |
| Giving preventive inoculations (except smallpox) | 26 | 92 |
| Performing venepuncture | 21 | 39 |
| Giving desensitising injections | 12 | 39 |
| Taking cervical smears | 9 | 39 |
| Incising boils/abscesses | 7 | 39 |
| Vaccinating against smallpox | 6 | 43 |
|  | (N = 81) | (N = 72) |

Source: B.L.E.C. Reedy, M. de Roumanie, D.J. Newell and M. Williams, 'The Nurses Working in Primary Medical Care in England' (Medical Care Research Unit, Newcastle upon Tyne, 1977).

Table 2: Changes in the Number and Location of First (New) Treatments Given by Health Authority-Employed Nurses in England 1972-5

| Location of Treatment: | New Treatments Given | | | | Percentage increase in New Treatments 1972-5 |
|---|---|---|---|---|---|
|  | 1972 | | 1975 | | |
|  | No. (thousands) | Per Cent | No. (thousands) | Per Cent | |
| In patients' homes | 1,060 | 59.5 | 1,119 | 48.0 | + 6 |
| In GP premises |  |  |  |  |  |
| Health centre | 192 | 10.8 ⎫ 40.5 | 497 | 21.3 ⎫ 52.0 | +159 |
| Other | 530 | 29.7 ⎭ | 717 | 30.7 ⎭ | + 35 |
| Totals | 1,782 | 100.0 | 2,333 | 100.0 | + 31 |

Source: Department of Health and Social Security, *Annual Report 1972* (London, HMSO, 1973); Department of Health and Social Security, Statistics and Research Division, personal communication (1977).

centres — which are known to be much more likely than other GP premises to have a special treatment room in which nurses can work.[5] As might be expected, the increase in the absolute number of first treatments in patients' homes was confined to those aged 65 or over, whereas in GP premises the increase occurred in all age groups but was most marked in those aged 5 to 64.

When taken in conjunction, these two sets of data provide circumstantial evidence that the impetus amongst health authority-employed nurses throughout the country is away from traditional care in the home and towards a more technical and 'medical' set of activities carried out with ambulant patients in the institutional setting of primary care premises. Thus it seems that the nurses employed by GPs were merely anticipating this movement amongst health authority-employed nurses and it is interesting to speculate how such a change of orientation amongst the latter might have been accelerated by the growth of health centres and by the development of 'attachment' and the concept of 'the team'.

At least in the community (if not necessarily in hospital), the implications for the emergence and use of auxiliaries and aides are clear. From a practical point of view it is important to know whether bedside care in the home will still be needed in the future and, second, whether the trend away from the bedside amongst professional nurses represents a permanent change in their ecology.

The first question is answered by the estimates of national growth in the proportion of the elderly in the population for the foreseeable future and the evidence from Table 2 confirms the experience of nursing administrators everywhere that the provision of home care for the elderly is a growing preoccupation for them.

The second question can be approached by a number of speculative explanations of the phenomenon which we are observing, and amongst them is the process of so-called 'professionalisation'. I suggest that we may also be observing a change of attitude and orientation towards their function amongst some 'attached' (health authority-employed) nurses. If so, then they seem to be identifying themselves increasingly with the objectives and methods of the physician as the other key member of the primary care team.

More pragmatically, I believe that this change is not only irreversible but will be progressive for the foreseeable future, with some community nurses reaching a high level of clinical autonomy in quasi-medical work. This will involve them particularly in the comparatively neglected elements of our health care system, which are those of health maintenance and the skilled long-term surveillance of chronic diseases. For this they will need prolonged and careful training similar to that provided for nurse practitioners in North America.

In conclusion: although the trend I have described does not 'explain' the existence and growth of aides and auxiliaries in the community nursing services, it does suggest that the two phenomena are linked in some way other than that of simple cause and effect. It also suggests that the people concerned cannot be considered in isolation from each other and that the fortunes of their auxiliaries and aides must become of real concern to the other members of the primary health care team.

## Notes

1. B.L.E.C. Reedy, P.R. Philips and D.J. Newell, 'Nurses and Nursing in Primary Medical Care in England', *British Medical Journal*, 2 (1976), pp.1304-6.
2. B.L.E.C. Reedy, M. de Roumanie,  D.J. Newell and M. Williams, 'The Nurses Working in Primary Medical Care in England' (Medical Care Research Unit, Newcastle upon Tyne, 1977).
3. Department of Health and Social Security, *Annual Report 1972* (London, HMSO, 1973).
4. Department of Health and Social Security, Statistics and Research Division, personal communication (1977).
5. D. Irvine and M. Jefferys, 'BMA Planning Unit survey of general practice, 1969', *British Medical Journal*, 4 (1971), pp.535-43.

# 8 EMPLOYEE PARTICIPATION IN THE CHANGE OF HOSPITAL ORGANISATION: EXPERIENCES WITH DEVELOPMENT OF A METHOD

Bjorg Elida Romedal (Norway)

**Summary**

What kind of changes does the staff in hospital want? And what will happen if their suggestions are put into action?

The Norwegian Institute for Hospital Research has worked with these questions. The main result of the project is the development of a method of problem-solving within the hospital. Stages of the method are:

(1) acclimatisation;
(2) interviews;
(3) analysis of data;
(4) discussions;
(5) experiments;
(6) evaluation;
(7) reports;
(8) diffusion.

The method does not revolutionise the hospital, at least in the short run. The method, however, seems to create critical attitudes in the staff, to clear up misunderstandings and to initiate a process of changing attitudes. Changes initiated from outside may be good enough, but radical changes also depend on the attitudes and motivation of the staff. These would only give good results if developed by the staff themselves.

**Introduction**

Examining hospitals as organisations is not an easy job, but it is a very interesting one. We find that hospitals are extremely complex organisations with many duties and tasks and with many different units and groups of workers. On the one hand you can say that hospitals are constantly changing with the introduction of new medical techniques and methods, new groups of specialists in different areas, new accounting routines, etc. On the other

179

hand, you can describe hospitals as stable organisations, laboriously developed over decades of experience and able to adapt to changes without developing destructive conflicts.

Today many people – inside as well as outside the hospital – show interest in the situation inside the hospital. And their questions are frustrating to people working within the system. I hope we can make use of the criticism in a positive way and not yield to the temptation to reject these discussions.

What kind of changes does the staff in hospital want? And what will happen if their suggestions are put into action?

**A Project**

Four years ago the results from a project at the Norwegian Institute for Hospital Research indicated that the staff in hospitals wanted to discuss their working situations. As a result, we began a study in 1974 at the University Hospital in Trondheim. Its aim was to analyse co-operation and to bring forward staff proposals for change.

We are convinced that people outside the hospitals may contribute with proposals and various good ideas. The hospital staff, however, know the situation and they have to make the ideas work. Permanent alterations depend on the staff's feeling of need for changes. Their motivation is also of vital importance. In addition, permanent alterations have to do with the staff's attitudes toward change in general.

The project aimed at:

increasing our knowledge of the life in hospitals in general and specifically in ward units;
looking more closely into different factors influencing co-operation;
using our experience to develop a method for problem-solving.

Two nurses, one sociologist and one social economist have been engaged in the project work.

We gained our experience from an orthopaedic and a medical ward at the University Hospital in Trondheim. Now we are going to test the results at a smaller hospital outside the town. At the same time we are working on a study related to the co-operation between the ward units and some service departments.

We acquired ideas from the Rowbottom study, described in the process report on the Brussels health services in London, 1973, even though this method was not quite appropriate for our purpose. We also acquired some ideas from modern organisational development studies in industry. Not much corresponding work seems to have been done in hospital organisations.

## The Method

A summary of the method follows here, with comment on the various steps. In practice, the different stages overlapped each other.

### Stage 1. Acclimatisation

This phase includes introduction, participation in the work and observations. Before we started, the staff was informed and accepted participation in the project. We were present at the ward on all shifts and got to know each other well. We found this stage an important one for developing mutual trust, which is an indispensable condition for the success of the project. We also learned a lot about how the staff look at their working situation.

### Stage 2. Interviews

Using the information obtained from the first stage, we developed an interview guide. We interviewed the entire staff, including part-time personnel. The interviews, lasting approximately one to two hours, gave us information about the employee's point of view on most aspects of the working situation. The topics covered are listed on p.184.

We used the same questions to all groups of employees participating in the interviews. The members of staff were also given the opportunity to comment on other relevant questions. The interviews were time-consuming and extensive, and we recommend a simpler questionnaire for the future, a questionnaire that may also be used during the evaluation stage.

You may ask whether interviews are necessary in addition to participant observation. Our answer is 'Yes.' This answer is based on the fact that the two different stages gave complementary information and also increased the validity and reliability of the study.

### Stage 3. Analysis of Data

This stage included the use of computers in the analysis of our data, but we also wrote a short report based on the data; to increase the staff's motivation for reading the report, it was made as informal as possible.

## Stage 4. Discussions

First, we had discussions with each staff group, commenting on the contents of the report and also ranking the different problems. Then we discussed each problem with the groups raising it. We discussed various ideas given in the interviews or taken up during the meeting. Some problems were dismissed as insoluble. For others we tried to find solutions that all the participants could accept. We held about thirty sessions in all. We regarded this stage as very important. It gives the staff an opportunity to look upon their situation from a critical point of view. They also get practice in problem formulation and discussion. The discussion sessions are also important because they provide opportunities for different groups to come together and become acquainted with each other and with the other group's problems. Misunderstandings were cleared up and proposals for new methods of work and co-operation were given. Some of these were tried out at a later stage. In summary, the employees gave preference to minor daily problems when proposing changes. Few proposals were related to more radical changes of the hospital structure and organisation.

Why? There is no certain answer but I shall suggest possibilities.

Nearly all employees are educated within the hospital. They have learned to know this special system and no others. From where can they obtain revolutionary ideas? The work-load is also great. Can we expect people working under such circumstances to have time and strength to develop new ideas and see their own situation objectively and as a part of a greater system? Generally, people also have difficulties in imagining situations qualitatively different from what they are used to.

Our conclusion on this point is that people outside the hospital with different background and experience may be of great help to the hospital staff in supplying fresh ideas and unorthodox points of view. It is of vital importance, however, that the employees themselves appraise the ideas and evaluate their practical value.

## Stage 5. Experiments

The staff problems discussed in the previous stage were not the same for the two ward units and the experiments tried out were also different. (A summary of experiments is given on p.184.) This experience supports our presumption that it is rarely possible to find general solutions to special problems. And nearly all problems taken up in our two ward units were special because of the different groups of patients, the personnel, the different tasks, the different physical environment, etc.

The staff decided in advance how long the experiment should go on. It was fully possible to make changes within the experimental period. With a few exceptions, the experiments were given a positive evaluation by the staff.

## Stage 6. Evaluation

The evaluation covered several points: first, changes in the staff's apprehension of their own working situation; next, highlighted important factors related to co-operation; and finally, testing the effect of the practical experiments.

For this evaluation, we used notes from our earlier observations and re-interviewing of the staff.

## Stage 7. Reports

This project has lasted for four years. We therefore have chosen to make several reports, to get continuous feedback from the hospital staff as well as from health authorities and also to sum up the knowledge acquired during the project. We have found this feedback very useful.

## Stage 8. Diffusion

After the evaluation the staff was free to make permanent new routines that were developed through the experimental period. The director of the hospital and leader of different groups were continuously informed and gave their support to the experiments.

Several results from the experimental period have been adapted by other ward units. In this process the leaders' part is very important.

Ideally, we might expect that the process we have initiated would go on without assistance from people outside the staff. We do not, however, count on this. An adviser was therefore appointed to the hospital to continue the project in other ward units and to bring fresh ideas to the staff.

## Conclusion

The main result of the project is the development of a method of problem-solving within the hospital. Here I have concentrated on describing this method, because I think this is the part of the project that will be of greatest general interest. The findings of the project are listed on p.185.

## Contents of Interviews

Personnel data
Working hours
Salary scales
Physical environment
Role expectations
Prestige
Influence over working situation
The information system
Co-operation
Management
Personal development
Division of labour
Amount of work

## Experiments

Employees gave preference to minor daily problems when proposing changes. Only few proposals were related to more radical changes of the hospital structure and organisation. Examples of experiments:

Introduction of team-work
Introduction of secretary in in-patient accommodation
Co-operation between practical nurses and nurses' aides
Timing of doctor's visit to the patients
Co-operation between physiotherapists and nurses
Co-operation between ergotherapists and nurses
Co-operation between social workers and nurses
Building changes
Patient transport to department of ergotherapy
Change in routines of giving medicine
Better information to the nurses' aides
List of furniture in in-patient accommodation
Common meeting
Nurses cardex
Communication between nurses and doctors
Ambulant therapy for day-patients (in Norway we do not have special 'day-patient wards')
Co-operation between nurses in hospital and nurses in the districts

Co-operation between in-patient accommodation and service departments

## Some Results and Experiences

Co-operation in the ward unit was characterised as good by 75-90 per cent of the personnel.

Good co-operation seemed to depend on the staff's possibilities to:

exert influence on their own working situation;
get information;
work independently;
put their competence into practice;
learn more (nearly 50 per cent wanted to learn more);
feel that they have an interesting job.

Our measurements also showed correlation between these aspects. A heavy work-load influenced co-operation in a negative way. The co-operation between registered nurses and practical nurses was good. There were few open conflicts and not many employees were willing to admit power as an aspect in conflict situations. In the hospital, employers as well as employees seem to believe in problem-solving by means of goodwill. In the hospital, most of the employees were women. Here we seem to have one of the reasons why the hospital is a stable organisation, an organisation with little articulated displeasure and few open conflicts. In order to increase the staff's possibility of having a say in management, the hospital practised decentralised boards in each unit as an experiment. In asking each employee if they knew their own representative, however, we found that about 80 per cent did not know of this experiment.

Different professional groups had different concepts of the notion of health. This fact complicated co-operation as well as communication and was also a reason for role conflicts. Ergotherapists, physiotherapists and, especially, social workers had the greatest role conflicts and also the greatest co-operation problems. These groups, and also some of the nurses, felt that there was little correspondence between the importance of their work and their relative prestige.

Because of the great work-load, the nurses had a constant feeling of guilt. The working situation does not permit them to fulfill their own expectations.

Thirty per cent of the staff wanted others to take over some of their duties. On in-patient accommodation the nurses wanted, and got, an assistant for office work placed in their in-patient accommodation.

On the other in-patient accommodation they received help for some office routines from outside. Both the in-patient accommodations gave their practice a good evaluation.

Service departments were influencing the working routines in the ward unit to a considerable extent and complicated the organisation of the work. In changes and diffusion, the engagement of leaders of different groups was of great importance. To support diffusion from one ward to the other the example of the staff was also very important.

Permanent changes often demanded changes of attitudes. Making changes, therefore, was, and ought to be, time-consuming.

Changes initiated from the outside may be good enough, but radical changes will only give good results if developed by the staff themselves. The hospitals as organisations are extremely complex and really contain *several* organisations.

In-patient accommodations are different because of different groups of patients, different groups of personnel, different medical techniques, different physical environment, etc. These different circumstances make it necessary for the special in-patient accommodation to find its special way for organising the work and co-operation. Generalising the problems and their solutions can hardly be recommended beyond a certain level.

## Bibliography

Axelsen, T. *Det tause sykehuset.* Universitetsforlaget, Oslo, 1976

Borum, F. *Organisation, makt og forandring.* Nyt Nordisk forlag, Köbenhavn, 1976

Heydebrand, W.V. *Hospitals Bureaucracy. A comparative study of organisations.* Punellen, New York, 1973.

Katz, D. and Kahn, R.L. *The Social Psychology of Organisations.* Weley, New York, 1966

Romedal, B.E. og Karlsen, S. *Funksjonsfordeling i helseinstitusjoner.* Rapport fra en sykepost – problemer og endringsforsøk. Delrapport II og III. STF81 A76009, STF81 A76015. Trondheim, 1976

Rowbottom, R. Hospital Organisation. A process report on the Brussel Health Services. London, 1973

Shortell, S.M. and Brown, M. (eds.). *Organisational Research in Hospital.* An Inquiry Book. Blue Cross Association, Chicago, 1976.

Thorsrud, E. og Emery, F.E. *Mot en ny bedriftsorganisasjon. Tanum,* Oslo, 1970

# 9 HOSPITAL STAFFING: SUMMARY OF A PROJECT

Leif Sonkin (Finland)

The definition of the number and structure of positions in a hospital
and its different working units is one of the most important of both
traditional and still opportune tasks of hospital administration. In
recent years the importance of the task has, however, become more
pronounced with differentiation of the hospital activities and with
increased central services. On the other hand, absenteeism and lack of
personnel have made it necesssary to study separately the positions
and personnel required.

So far, head nurses have been in charge of planning the nursing staff,
but the factors mentioned above have made them look for different
facilities in the planning task that has become exceedingly difficult.
Thus, the Finnish Hospital League has formed a project to study both
basic staffing and the day-to-day personnel allocation in a hospital.
This report is the first of two reports and deals with a method for
defining the need of positions – a method which in turn strives to apply
general principles of generally approved methods of work analysis,
bearing in mind the level of precision and the special demands of
health care.

The purpose of the recommendation is to assist hospitals and health
centres to dimension the staff on wards, medical services departments
and administrative and technical units in a more exact and objective
way, as well as to assist them in their efforts to achieve a more practical
usage of the personnel resources they have. The report is intended to
be used by head nurses, head physicians, personnel secretaries,
planning secretaries, administrators and work groups
participating in the planning process. The report can also be
used in training health care personnel.

The recommendation shows how the activities and work
organisation of the hospital and its various working units have to be
planned in order to calculate the number and structure of positions
that the patients and the technical level and other special characteristics
of the hospital require. It is also possible to use the method in estimating
which objectives can be reached if the number of positions and
personnel are given and if there is a lack of personnel.

The method is based on studying the work carried out in the

hospital, on dividing it into parts, and on rearranging it so that the work input required can be estimated. Planning is essentially based on the work of the hospital's own personnel, and only in the beginning will the assistance and guidance of the Finnish Hospital League be needed.

The method has been applied in defining the positions of nursing and assisting personnel in the wards and medical service departments of the Seinäjoki Central Hospital. The results have been encouraging.

With this method, hospitals and health centres can also ease the personnel situation in the whole country by studying and if needed by changing their personnel structure in a carefully considered way. The method can also be used to make the study on personnel structure which is needed for the national five-year plan (1978-82).


Reprinted from Finnish Hospital League Bulletin.

# PART FOUR: DISCUSSION SUMMARIES

# GROUP 1: TRAINING

Chairman: Mr E.R. Pyne
Rapporteur: Miss J. Tinch

Within the group's membership were those who are providing, supervising and planning such training in a variety of countries and of areas within the United Kingdom. We agreed that where nursing auxiliaries are implied, it is necessary to provide instruction for them. This instruction should be provided by and within the employing organisation. It should be compulsory and should preferably be given prior to starting practical work. While waiting for an appointment on an instruction course, prospective employees might be encouraged to prepare themselves by attending, for example, a British Red Cross Society home nursing course. This would give them some opportunity to practise skills they would be learning at greater length later on and get some idea of the work that is involved in nursing.

There was agreement that a common core of instruction should be given to all nursing auxiliaries. This could be taken with other appropriate categories of staff in whole or in part. The common core should be about two weeks' duration or equivalent and it should introduce the course members (1) to the organisation in which they will work, and (2) to the duties which they will undertake. During this period the employee should be helped to set further learning targets in relation to his job description, as well as to recognise the limits and consequences of such duties. A variety of teaching methods, including demonstration and practice of skills, should be used. By the end of this two-week period the employee should know his terms and conditions of service, the scope and limits of the service he would provide, the basic needs of people and the basic needs of patients, safe codes of conduct and the legal implications relative to the nature of his employment.

Training and achievement should be recorded. This includes a record of instruction given and of abilities shown. Over the subsequent two to three months a flexible on-the-job training programme based on the individual's job description should be followed. During this period practical skills will be developed under the supervision of qualified nurses. In addition, a planned study programme will be provided through teaching by appropriate staff by means of study periods. The progress of each individual should be assessed and his suitability for the job discussed with the individual during this period. Further training throughout an individual's career should be provided by means of study periods to meet the changing needs within the organisation, to introduce new methods, equipment and procedures, and to discuss nursing problems and standards of care. Instruction should be controlled by staff with an in-service training remit in accordance with the policy of the employing authority and within national guidelines. The nurse manager has responsibilities in relation to the organisation of the nursing auxiliaries as workers and as trainees, their deployment in accordance with their learned ability, and their learning needs.

We would stress the following points.

(1)    there should be a clear policy with regard to the responsibilities of nursing auxiliaries;
(2)    there should be an agreed policy within the employing authority regarding the implementation of training;
(3)    there should be a continuing record of instruction and abilities relative to the job description for each individual.

# GROUP 2: TEAM INTEGRATION

Chairman: Miss B. Hall
Rapporteur: Mr R.F. Fisher

Our subject was team integration, division of labour, ratios and duties related to other nurses in hospital and community environments. Our first task was to decide what the animal was we were supposed to discuss. The next question was: do we need it? After prolonged discussion we decided that (a) we have them; they exist and we cannot ignore the situation; and (b) yes, we do need them, and therefore we must do something about them and the existing situation. In fact, we decided that we require two levels of nurse, a three-year trained nurse, a one- to two-year trained nurse, and a helper. The helper is, of course, the nursing auxiliary.

We considered the nursing auxiliary in isolation, but it was felt that this was a position which we would not encourage. We really do not want another isolated or fragmented group of care staff who are without room to develop. In isolation we can only see a repeat performance of the current pantomime of operating department assistants or ODAs presently playing in a number of health districts within this country. It is felt that we should aim for the team approach in nursing, for example in the nursing care plan, with the nursing auxiliary as a member of that team in, for instance, the plumber's mate role. We did not reach this particular point without a lot of discussion. The nursing care plan should be created by the qualified nurse based on the dependency of the patient and should be carried out by the total team. The approach should not be task-orientated but would obviously include tasks. Integration of the nursing auxiliary into the team is seen as being of great importance and it is from there that we went on to discuss ratios.

Consideration of a ratio of nurses or team members to nursing auxiliaries is impossible if you attempt to talk about them on a national level. However, just as the dependency of the individual patient will determine the nursing care plan, so it will determine the ratio of nurses to nursing auxiliaries. The professional judgement of the qualified nurse in charge will determine the danger point below which the team cannot be allowed to function or to fall. Discussion of the team and its membership brought us to the point of talking about a generic auxiliary or an auxiliary who can function as an aide to all paramedical professions. This, we felt, was a topic which requires further discussion.

Other topics which we feel require further formal investigation are:

(1)    the extent to which team nursing is practised;
(2)    is the ideal of one nurse to one patient correct or in the best interest of the patient and nurse?
(3)    some sort of comparison of the effectiveness of different mixes within the nursing care team;
(4)    what are the economic results of the different mixes of staff in nursing care teams?

Our final consideration was of the nursing auxiliary in the community environment. Once more we saw or see the auxiliary as a member of the team. We were given the example of the nursing auxiliary based in the local hospital providing support for the community nurses in those situations where two pairs of hands are required, with the nursing auxiliary being available on demand. The use of the nursing auxiliary again will be determined by the dependency of the patients for whom one is providing a service. The service and assistance will in effect be that which would normally be provided by a relative if one were available.

# GROUP 3: SUPERVISION

Chairman: Miss B. Tierney
Rapporteur: Miss M. Yeo

Group 3's remit was supervision, patterns of supervision, relationships
and responsibilities, and professional and legal implications. This was
a very wide remit which seemed to overlap all the other groups. We
found that we were often talking about different people when we
talked about the nursing auxiliary. In the countries represented in
the group and from the information circulated, it is obvious that
there are a number of differences. It took a considerable time to agree
on the definition, as in the International Council of Nurses' Category
III nursing personnel definition.

The role most acceptable to the group was that of a member of
the nursing team functioning as an assistant to, rather than as a
substitute for, the nurse. From there we needed to define what was
meant by supervision, and this took considerable time. It was agreed
that supervision should be defined as an enabling process, a relationship
between people which has a special purpose, whereby the supervisor
enables the supervised to develop his or her individual abilities and to
acquire the skills needed to accomplish a defined, agreed and understood
objective. It was also seen to be a supportive function within the
organisational structure in which the nursing auxiliary is working.
Checkpoints needed to be established within that structure since the
quality and extent of supervision is directly related to the care and
attention received by the patient. Supervision is an important part of
the administrative process, i.e. the manager's responsibility.
Supervision and checkpoints have to be built into a clearly defined
programme of training. It is the nurse managers who must decide
what is needed at this level of work, basing their decisions on the
patients' needs. It should then be possible to lay down the areas in
which the nursing auxiliary will work and to agree appropriate
patterns of supervision. In the United Kingdom we decided that
these decisions must be taken locally to take account of the existing
situation but that national, area and professional policies, where these
exist, should also be taken into consideration.

After considering some of the tools required for effective
supervision, the role of job descriptions was discussed. There was

195

disagreement between those who wanted very clearly defined job descriptions and those who wanted them fairly flexible. We felt that they should clearly define the job but should not be rigidly task-orientated. Job descriptions should be constantly reviewed and some felt they should allow for a fair degree of flexibility.

Training programmes were not in our remit but cannot be divorced from supervision. Programmes should be linked with job descriptions. The recruitment and selection procedures should be planned to match the job with the job-holder and to prescribe tasks within the range of the competence of the individual. We also felt that continuous assessment should be carried out.

We looked at indicators of effective supervision but could reach no conclusion without an agreed definition of 'satisfactory care'. We felt that patient and relatives' satisfaction should be taken into account, as well as staff morale, including wastage, sickness and absence rates, overtime rates and various others. At this point time ran out.

In sum, we felt that supervision was part of the administrative process and the manager's responsibility at all levels. The team leader, a qualified nurse, is responsible for the overall nursing function. She can delegate tasks within that function but she cannot delegate responsibility for the function. She/he prescribes the various patterns of nursing care, assesses the needs and evaluates the results. The team leader is usually a qualified nurse, but in some of the countries represented in our group there was more than one level of nursing auxiliary. In that case the nursing auxiliary might then need to supervise another nursing auxiliary at a lower level. This was discussed, but no agreement could be reached.

If the grade of auxiliary is necessary, and not all members of the group seemed to be convinced of this, we decided that the profession must recognise this. A range of responsibility for the nursing auxiliary grade needs to be defined and training programmes designed to cover the needs. Nursing team leadership and supervisory skills need to be included in professional nurse training. In terms of legal implications there are problems in the UK, because apparently there is no case law to guide us. The comment from one country was that trained nurses have legal protection of name but not of function. Within Sweden, where the procedures have gone further, legal responsibility lies within the framework of training and education, but the degree to which these duties can be extended depends on the views of the person who delegates the task to the other person.

# GROUP 4: ORGANISATIONAL MODELS

Chairman: Professor J.E.F. Hastings
Rapporteur: Miss B.M. Stocking

The group, like the other groups, found it very difficult to separate the question of whether there was really a need for a nursing auxiliary from all the other factors which compound the issue: the current economic situation, fears about shortage of jobs for trained nurses and professional jealousies. We tried to put aside our biases and decide whether nursing auxiliaries were merely being employed because of expediency or whether, in fact, we would have to invent them if they did not exist.

Miss Lambert opened the discussion by presenting a paper in which she made a case for the restriction of nursing auxiliaries in terms of the numbers employed, in the work they carried out, and in the use of the title nurse. In part our group's conclusion agreed with this. It was felt that reduction in numbers was needed and there was a strong feeling that in some situations the ratio of qualified nurses to auxiliaries was out of joint, with the auxiliaries being given too much responsibility. We felt it was essential to define the work of the auxiliary and to provide whatever training is necessary.

The group also felt that there should be a reduction in the numbers and activities of auxiliaries but definitely not an extinction of the nursing auxiliary. We did conclude that auxiliaries would have to be invented if they did not exist. We agreed that their function was greater in the area of basic nursing care but that a range of technical functions might also be carried out by auxiliaries trained in the necessary skills and appropriately supervised. It was pointed out to our group that talking about skills does not equate at all with talking about the level of work or the level of responsibility that someone is capable of taking. Although we felt that auxiliaries can make a special contribution, we found it hard to agree on what that special contribution was. It was suggested that auxiliaries were carrying out the nursing that a relative might otherwise do, that the auxiliary had time, particularly time to talk, and had a special contribution to make because she was well accepted by the patient. Thus the auxiliary may provide what Professor Hastings called 'a sort of mothering function' which may nevertheless require some

197

training, to understand the stresses of illness and the basic nursing care required.

Although these comments were accepted as valid, this went very little way towards sorting out the confusion about what auxiliaries should be doing. To analyse this further, we moved on to look at the organisational settings in which auxiliaries are working. We recognise that the employment of auxiliaries in hospitals and in the community are quite different, in part because of different legal responsibilities; perhaps more important, however, because of the ease of access of staff to one another in the hospital and the continual observation of the patient in the hospital setting. In other words, the hospital itself provides a sort of protection for the employment of the auxiliary which does not exist as strongly in the community. We began by thinking about the community setting and agreed that auxiliaries can play a useful role in the community in relation to nursing. This is also true of other auxiliaries in relation to other professionals. We felt that the role should be one of being an assistant to the nurse and that this is a very important role in the health team. The auxiliary should be under a close degree of supervision by the nurse and there should clearly be set limits to the amount of discretion given to the auxiliary. We recognised, however, that there are extremely capable, intelligent auxiliaries who for one reason or another cannot complete nurse training as it now stands, and who might be able to take more responsibility.

Our conclusion was that the amount of supervision an auxiliary needed should be left to the professional judgement of the supervising nurse based on the capability of the auxiliary. In the community it is particularly important that this supervision and back-up by other professionals is available.

In hospitals we recognise that there are some circumstances, such as intensive care units, where it may not be appropriate to use auxiliaries at all; that even in one ward it may be appropriate that an auxiliary give a bed-bath to one patient but not to another. This led us to a more general formulation of the auxiliary's role. There are normal patient needs, feeding, bathing, etc., and where they do differ greatly from what the patient would require if he were not ill, these can be delegated to an auxiliary. Over and above this there are special instances where these normal needs should be taken care of by a professional and special technical needs related to the patient's illness where the professional skill is also called for. There are tasks then that by and large will be done by a qualified nurse. There are other tasks which by and large will be done by an auxiliary. As with the auxiliary in the community, it is the need for supervision by the qualified nurse and delegation by the qualified nurse which distinguishes the auxiliary from the professional.

Thus, although we began by saying that the hospital and the community were quite different, we reached a sort of common conclusion that the essence is that the auxiliary should be supervised by the professional and that the professional should delegate to the auxiliary. This has implications for nursing education. It is essential that the professional nurse realises that they have the final responsibility and also that they have to provide supervision and delegation and we need to change some attitudes towards this. Perhaps this should be done in nursing education itself. It was also recognised that it is the nurse who has responsibility for motivating and encouraging the auxiliary. The conclusions that we came to about accountability of the auxiliary hold true for many other professions and groups inside and outside the Health Service.

This led us on to thinking about the future and how our model of the auxiliary's role could fit into it. Our friends from other countries led us in thinking about this as we began to question whether we needed an auxiliary in a whole variety of professions or whether a broader type of helping person was not feasible. An auxiliary who is an amalgamation of home help and nursing auxiliary already exists in Sweden. Canada has a similar person in the human services model in some provinces. In the Netherlands there have been experiments with a combined home help and nursing auxiliary in maternity care. It seemed to us to be of much greater benefit to the individual receiving help if, instead of the fragmented service that we provide now, a similar sort of generic person could be used in the United Kingdom. I was interested to see that Group 2 also came to a similar conclusion. Instead of looking vertically and seeing a helper in each profession we need to look horizontally, to provide one person who could be the point of access to a number of services. We need to look at the individuals who will be providing this generic function. They will have different levels of capability and we must have the flexibility so that these people can be used as fully as possible.

One topic came up several times in our discussion, fundamental to the whole. This is the issue of whether we are not over-helping individuals. We question the extent to which the community or the state should take on the responsibility for the health, health maintenance and social welfare of its members and whether individuals could not be encouraged to play a greater role in responsibility for their own health. We recognise that this could not take place overnight, and it would require the initiatives of the health professionals to help people achieve this greater degree of responsibility. Nevertheless, as Katherine Elliott puts it, 'In the final analysis we are all health workers.'

# SUMMATION OF WORKSHOP

## Rapporteur: Professor A. Altschul

I begin with a few personal comments, because this may help you to see more clearly to what extent I too am subject to forces which cause selective perception and which result in the introduction of value judgement and bias. I have been unable in the course of this workshop to understand how the specific people came to be here, how the specific participants and the groups of participants came together. I think there was clearly an assumption that the problems which the researchers have uncovered in Britain do exist to some extent in other countries, but I am not sure whether participants came because they have problems or because they have solved the problems. I have become aware that even within the United Kingdom the size and the nature of the problems are situation-specific, so what do we take away from this conference? How are we going to apply the more generalised conclusions to the specific interests which each of us has in a subject?

Did we assemble here to try and resolve the problems by pooling our diverse experiences? The brief that you received from me on the first day suggested that. My question then was, how can we continue to collaborate and implement good ideas and practices? I think there was an assumption that we had good ideas, otherwise we would not be able to put them into action. I further enquired whether there were any practical suggestions for consulting each other, suggestions in which the Nursing Research Unit and the International Hospital Federation could lend support. Could we consider alternative models and could we suggest practical examples?

I do think we stayed fairly close to the brief and many practical ideas were suggested. But I am not clear who was trying to help whom. I believe we all felt a little threatened and inclined to assume that each one of us was all right really. It was only the others who needed the help. This led to a holding back, a failure of people to give others the benefit of the detailed description and analysis of the issues we were taking for granted. It took time before we cleared up whether we wanted auxiliaries, whether we wanted to use them better, more effectively and more efficiently, or whether we really

201

preferred not to have them at all. This came up again in almost every group report today.

Some of us took it for granted that we were talking of untrained people in speaking of the auxiliary, but others do not have this idea at all. The latter failed to comprehend how any of the former could have got themselves into this untutored situation in the first place. Some took it for granted that we knew all about the proper function of the qualified nurse and that we were only worried about the auxiliaries. But, when challenged, we could not really decide whether we all agreed about the nature of nursing work itself. Some of the time we assumed that qualified nurses did a good job but at other times we were despondent even about this particular idea.

We did agree that the chief virtue of the auxiliary is her humanity, her ability to listen, to have empathy, to have spare time. This is extremely depressing in the implications that it has for nurses. We were confronted with the truth that many of us were reluctant to share our nursing function with  less well-qualified people. We said that if we did have to use auxiliaries at least we wanted to keep them firmly in a subordinate role.

Yesterday, Mrs Pereira reinforced this attitude and she gave us a dire warning. She said 'It is dangerous to give auxiliaries some training!' When we do this they end up by wanting even more and they are actually really wanting to become nurses. Very dangerous indeed! She gave us a marvellous example of the Portuguese experience, in which there were successive waves of unrest. We realised that in the United Kingdom we had heard all this before, twelve years ago when we assimilated auxiliaries into the State Enrolled category. Will we still be saying the same thing in twelve years' time?

We were also asked to try and think about whether indeed we can care for people at all if we do not care for each other sufficiently to recognise each other's talents. I think on this somewhat sad but also challenging topic we were given the tone for the workshop by Dr Elliott. On this theme she spread before us a wide canvas of inefficiency and helplessness in the face of world-wide suffering and poverty, and she pointed out to us all the dilemmas which arise when we consider the lack of 'fit' of our elegant training to the inelegant settings 'in which to use it'. She also optimistically showed us the direction in which we should move to be, again her words, 'on tap', and she urged us to find a way in which each worker in a team can make maximum contributions at his own level of competence and can assume maximum responsibility and accountability in his own allowable discretionary space. Dr Elliott asked us to examine whether the lessons learned from developing countries could conceivably have any applications in Western countries. But I do not think that we resolved whether any of the sixteen or so countries here represented could be exempt from the label of 'developing country'.

Groups were asked to discuss issues about auxiliaries in relation to four topics. In practice, it was found difficult to draw clear lines between each group's topic and that of others. In the group reports the particular issue was properly highlighted, but others were touched on at the same time. Mr Sonkin made the point most clearly, that we need to discuss these issues in the form of a feedback loop. He showed us several diagrams which started at different positions, and returned after moving through the whole, i.e. organisation, training, supervision, back to organisation. Other speakers also referred to the need to assess the total situation within which the problem of the auxiliary is to be discussed. None did so more clearly than Lisbeth Hockey, who left us in no doubt at all that professional matters, economics and politics must be inextricably linked. I shall try to sum up under the same headings as your group discussion reports.

## Training

Mr Hardie collated from your papers the length of training which you offered to various grades and participating nations, and categorised it in terms of years or months. I looked at this also in terms of hours. We range from 415 to 510 hours in Norway, 185 in Austria, 300 in Denmark, approximately 200 in Switzerland and Sweden, but I have also heard one of the groups talk about 4 to 6 hours in Britain. Some background papers highlighted theoretical instruction. France, on the other hand, did not specify the content of training and others, like Belgium and Switzerland, emphasised the essentially practical in-service nature of the preparation. Examinations were mentioned by Germany and Canada, however, with no detail. Others left it either wide open or expressed doubt about the possibility of finding a suitable method of assessing competence in the course of training. Of the background statements you produced, the Norwegian was the most detailed but also the most candid in admitting freely that the whole situation is still very confused. There are still many unqualified auxiliaries, and this was mentioned from Belgium, Canada, Germany, Switzerland and from Spain, where this applied until fairly recently. Only the Dutch claim to have no auxiliaries at all.

I think all groups agreed that there should be some compulsory instruction. The question of whether health auxiliaries have enough of a common core of work to allow for collective training was mentioned in all sessions. The idea of having a generic auxiliary is of course as attractive as the idea of a generic social worker was, and as the idea of a generic nurse sometimes appears to some people. My own point about this, however, is that wherever generic training has been put into operation, people begin to specialise just a few years later. This is because, in fact, you cannot operate generically; you can only operate specifically.

A point that was raised is the idea of a record of instruction and abilities. As I listened to you, I thought back about the little booklet nurses used to carry around with them in which they were meant to have a record of instruction. I am sure I am not the only one who remembers how this was finally filled in, so whether there is any possibility of putting a record of instruction for auxiliaries into operation, I do not know. Is it not likely that the record of instruction would tell us more about the supervisor than about the person who is being instructed? Was it suggested, though I did not hear it, that we would in fact discharge a person who failed to reach the required standards? I am very glad it will never be my particular responsibility.

**Team Integration**

On this theme the papers gave very interesting details which were nevertheless very difficult to compare. For example, some countries listed several types of aides, four in Austria and Finland, but these do not have the same or equivalent names. It was difficult to see to what extent common training or common usage would be possible. Others referred to the quality of team integration difficult for some, more promising for others. Some of you stated whether there are legal implications to the level of accountability or responsibility that each team member has.

We must thank Muriel Skeet for the help she gave us in conceptualising the different team structures in which we can operate. She gave us different models of shared responsibility and of division of labour. She also reminded us that untrained relatives and friends are the largest group of helpers and that they need support, instruction and guidance from the professional. Dr Stewart's and Mrs Hawker's joint paper spelt this out again and emphasised the need for team co-ordination: 'All the different tasks and accomplishments are part of a whole to whose product all in some degree contribute.'

It was proposed that we need nurses of three-year training, some of two-year training, and helpers. Of course, it is the helpers about whom we have spent these days cogitating. But, about the helpers, there were more caveats than there were prescriptions for use. We must think of danger points. We must think of ratios. We must think about the usefulness of a generic auxiliary. We must differentiate between the usage in a community team and the usage in various other situations within hospitals or homes. We were told that there are certain tasks where we must have two pairs of hands. On those occasions we ought to be able to call on the help of an assistant who ought then to be 'on tap', I suppose, whenever we want her. My rather irreverent thought went to the time when my house was being rewired. The electrician who was working all alone said to me one morning, 'I must get a move on. I must finish all the things I can do by myself by Thursday, because on Thursday I have an apprentice. That is when I will do all the jobs for which I need another pair of hands.' Now what exactly the apprentice learned, which is worth learning, and how the auxiliary learns if she is only an extra pair of hands, I am not clear about.

**Supervision**

This topic was rather thin in background papers. However, the question of what the ratio between the qualified and others ought to be has clearly got significance for supervision. Belgium, for example, has a 7 to 3 ratio whereas Sweden has 32,000 trained against 52,000 auxiliaries, a totally different ratio. This kind of range reflects exactly the kind of range between nations which Melissa Hardie has already found within Britain. Norway told us it was approximately 50-50, Denmark has 2,300 nurses and 4,000 assistants. It is difficult to draw any conclusions from these figures in that not all of you mentioned students. Some did, and some said that students were not counted as learners, therefore were separately supervised. Some said that students form part of the work-force and therefore must be supervised. How many auxiliaries a trained person can supervise must depend to some extent on how many students the same person supervises. I could not get that kind of figure from your reports. Only France said that all *aides soignantes* are completely supervised; I would be interested to find out how this is in fact done. In the plenary discussions we frequently touched on worries and anxieties which nurses experience about moral responsibilities and about their legal accountability when what may be defined as nursing tasks are delegated to those with lesser skills.

Mr Cang was the speaker who for me provided what I can only describe as an 'Aha!' experience. My field of vision changed completely and my thought processes made a big leap when the concepts he spoke about fell into place. I do not know if any of you have read a book called *Mr God this is Anna?* That book did something like it to me in suddenly switching my entire perspective. Of course, we were speaking all the time of two levels of work which differ in the amount of discretion the workers can use and the different degree of prescription attached to the task.

Group 3 indicated that improved recruitment and selection and planned and prescribed job descriptions might help us in continuous assessment of the staffing state of affairs. It was said that the national policies must be taken into account at the local level. Do we know how exactly in any particular setting where to interpret national standards? Group 3 did want to think about all staff groups at the same time and about the generic kind of assistant which might help everyone. They made the interesting point that if we could find indices of high morale we would also automatically learn something about the relationships between nurses and their helpers.

### Organisational Models

Organisation, supervision and training hang together. This aspect was most fully documented in the papers, which not only give us the present picture, but also show how it has developed, and in which direction different countries are hoping to go. Finland, for example, with their five-year plan, which is annually adjusted, was very helpful in aiding us to visualise the organisation. Austria says they are currently reducing the number of auxiliaries, Belgium is giving auxiliaries paid educational leave to become nurses, Germany has plans to have training for all but finds it 'difficult to achieve this'. Interesting was the paper from Holland — it should be read in detail because it provides reasons why it has no auxiliaries. Could it apply to our own situation?

The recurrent thought is the one I have already mentioned, 'Do we use auxiliaries as an expediency or are they really needed?' Melissa Hardie proposed this dilemma. Her paper, I think, suggests that we all need them. Mr Johnson's very beautiful paper also covered this ground from a different viewpoint, that of a sociologist with particular knowledge and expertise at looking at social phenómena. Professional jealousies, a case for restriction of numbers, but always with the rider that we do not want to lose them altogether. This was said loudly and clearly by the report stating that we do not want the extinction of the auxiliary, we only want to restrict them. Do I recall something like that happening in medical schools in regard to the number of doctors they were willing to train? When we get to a stage where we are going to control the entry to the profession in the way the printers do, I would be very careful about who may or may not come in, in the first instance. Group 4 again touched on training and highlighted the desirability of the generic social worker but, of course, with the final conclusion that we already have generic social workers. Each one of us is such a generic social worker because we all are health professionals.

We leave this workshop heavier by several pounds of food and paper, and we leave on a higher level of confusion, but we have made new contacts, perhaps new friends. I think we will leave with a new determination to tackle the enormous problems which were the subject of our thinking. Personally, I leave with renewed optimism about the chances of success.

# LIST OF CONTRIBUTORS

*Katherine Elliott*, Assistant Director, Ciba Foundation, London, England

*Melissa Hardie*, Research Associate, Nursing Research Unit, University of Edinburgh, Edinburgh, Scotland

*Miles Hardie*, Director General, International Hospital Federation, London, England

*Margaret Hawker*, Superintendent Physiotherapist, Department of Geriatric Medicine, Edgware General Hospital, Edgware, Middlesex, England

*Lisbeth Hockey*, Director, Nursing Research Unit, University of Edinburgh, Edinburgh, Scotland

*Malcolm L. Johnson*, Lecturer, Nuffield Centre for Health Services Studies, University of Leeds, Leeds, Yorkshire, England

*David Rye*, Director of Professional Activities, Royal College of Nursing, London, England

*Muriel Skeet*, Chief Nursing Officer, British Red Cross, London, England

*Monnica Stewart*, Assistant Physician, Department of Geriatric Medicine Edgware General Hospital, Edgware, Middlesex, England

*Stephen Cang*, Convenor, Health Services Organisation Research Unit, Brunel University, Uxbridge, Middlesex, England

*Margaret Irvine*, Chief Administrative Nursing Officer, Northern Health and Social Services Board, Northern Ireland

*Morag Lambert*, Senior Nursing Officer – In-service Education, Greater Glasgow Health Board, Glasgow, Scotland

*Norman S. Martin*, Honorary General Secretary and Founder, Nursing Auxiliaries Association, Cranleigh, Surrey, England

*Maria T.Q. Pereira*, Ministry of Social Affairs, Lisbon, Portugal

*M.E.F. Perkins*, Area Nurse – Service Planning, West Sussex Area Health Authority, Worthing, Sussex, England

*Barry L.E.C. Reedy*, Senior Lecturer, Organisation of Health Care, Medical Care Research Unit, University of Newcastle-upon-Tyne, England

*Bjorg Elida Romedal*, Research Officer, Norwegian Institute for Hospital Research, Trondheim, Norway

*Leif Sonkin*, The Finnish Hospital League, Helsinki, Finland

# LIST OF PARTICIPANTS

*Miss B.A. Adams*, Senior Nursing Officer – Clinical Management Assignments, Birmingham Health District (Central)

*Mr W.J. Allen*, Nursing Officer, Department of Health and Social Services, Belfast, Northern Ireland

*Miss M.G. Auld*, Chief Nursing Officer, Scottish Home and Health Department, Edinburgh

*Miss M.L. Badouaille*, National Group Work Leader in Continuing Education, Paris, France

*Mrs E. Barnes*, Education Secretary, Norsk Hjelpepleierforbund, Oslo, Norway

*Miss L. Barton*, Registered Nursing Assistant, Toronto, Canada

*Sr M.J. Berchmans*, Matron, Mater Maternity Hospital, Dublin, Ireland

*Mr W. Black*, Nursing Officer, Northern Health and Social Services Board, Ballymena, Northern Ireland

*Miss A. Bonner*, Divisional Nursing Officer, Ilford, Essex

*Mrs P. Borley*, Nursing Officer, Crewe, Cheshire

*Miss M.P. Bull*, District Nursing Officer, Swansea Health District, Swansea, Wales

*Miss B. Byrne*, Nursing Officer – Manpower Planning, Scottish Home and Health Department, Edinburgh

*Dr C. Cerquella*, Director, Advanced College of Nursing, Madrid, Spain

*Miss I. Cook*, District Physiotherapist, Lewisham, London

*Mr H.R. Cruddace*, Area Nurse – Service Planning, Sunderland Area Health Authority

*Miss M.F. Cullen*, Nurse Administrator, Health Advisory Service (NHS), England

*Miss M.A. Day*, District Nursing Officer, Tower Hamlets Health District, London

*Mr R.F. Fisher*, Regional Nurse, South East Thames Regional Health Authority, Croydon, Surrey

*Mrs M.E. Furbank*, Nursing Officer, Liskeard, Cornwall

*Miss S.A.G. Garrett*, Senior Tutor, King's Fund College, London

*Mrs W. Gavelin*, Scientific Officer, Swedish Planning and Research

Institute (SPRI), Stockholm

*Miss M.H. Gilmore*, Regional Nursing Officer, East Anglian Regional Health Authority, Cambridge

*Miss A.S. Grant*, Education Officer, Central Midwifery Board for Scotland, Edinburgh

*Miss P. Guyer*, Senior Nursing Officer – Personnel, Northwick Park Hospital and Clinical Research Centre, Harrow

*Mrs I. Gyde-Petersen*, National Secretary, Dansk Kommunal Arbejderforbund, Copenhagen, Denmark

*Miss B. Hall*, Regional Nursing Officer, West Midlands Regional Health Authority, Birmingham

*Mr St J.V. Hall*, Regional Nurse, Professional Education and Development, North Yorkshire

*Prof J.E.F. Hastings*, Associate Dean, Community Health, University of Toronto, Canada

*Miss M. Hofer*, Nursing Section, Schweiz Krankenhausinstitut Aarau, Switzerland

*Miss J.C. Hope*, Senior Nursing Officer, The Royal Infirmary, Edinburgh

*Miss I. Johnsson*, Section Head, Department of Planning, National Board of Health and Social Welfare, Stockholm

*Mr D. Jones*, Sub-Area Nursing Officer, Gwynedd Area Health Authority Wales

*Mrs M. Jussari*, Head of Nursing Research Office, Turun Yliopispollinen Keskussairaata, Turku, Finland

*Miss G.M. Kirk*, In-service Education Officer, Bangour General Hospital, Broxburn, Scotland

*Miss I.B. Knight*, Chief Professional Adviser, Scottish Council for Health Education, Edinburgh

*Prof J.D.E. Knox*, Department of General Practice, University of Dundee Scotland

*Miss E. Kristiansen*, Director of Nursing Services, Central Hospital of Rogaland, Stavanger, Norway

*Dr E.V. Kuenssberg*, President, Royal College of General Practitioners, and general practitioner, West Granton Medical Group, Edinburgh

*Mrs P. Lyytikäinen,* Planner, The Finnish Hospital League, Helsinki

*Miss S. Macrae*, Area Nursing Officer (Personnel), Tayside Health Board, Dundee, Scotland

*Miss O.M. McLeod*, Nursing Officer, Royal Infirmary, Glasgow

*Mrs P. Manock*, Health Visitors' Association, London

*Mrs M.I. Martin*, Area Nurse (Personnel), Aylesbury, Bucks., England

*Mr A. Mitchell*, Area Nursing Officer, Barnsley Area Health Authority,

Barnsley, South Yorkshire
*Miss H.T. Mitchell*, Senior Nursing Officer — In-service Training,
  Southern General Hospital, Glasgow
*Miss A. Mukherjee*, Tutor, Royal College of Nursing, London
*Miss H.E. New*, Clinical Teacher of Nursing Auxiliaries, St
  Bartholomew's Hospital, London
*Mrs Y. Nielsen*, In-service Training Sister, Dudley Road Hospital, Birmingham
*Miss G. Nilson*, Director of Nursing, Orupssjukhuset, Höör, Sweden
*Mrs L. Orme*, Nursing Officer — Training, Bury St Edmunds,
  Suffolk
*Mr N.E. Oud*, Charge Nurse, Valerius Hilnieh Hospital, Amsterdam
*Miss J. Parry*, Senior Nursing Officer — Planning and Research,
  St James's University Hospital, Leeds
*Mrs B. Pettersson*, Head of Planning Section, The Federation of
  Swedish County Councils
*Oberin W.V. Poncet*, Johanniter-Schwesternschaft, Bonn
*Sr M.L. Power*, Chairman, Nursing Assistant Advisory Committee,
  Newfoundland, Canada
*Miss M. Prem*, Sister Tutor, Heppenheim, Germany
*Mr E.R. Pyne*, Senior Nursing Officer — Training, Orpington, Kent
*Dr A. Rolleder*, Public Health Officer, Federal Ministry of Health and
  Environmental Protection, Vienna, Austria
*Miss M. Rychtelska*, Nurse Adviser, International Council of Nurses,
  Geneva
*Miss O.E. Senior*, Regional Nursing Officer, Trent Regional Health
  Authority, Sheffield
*Mrs A. De Smet Simoens*, Inspectorate of Schools for Paramedical
  Personnel, Brussels, Belgium
*Mrs M. Sjostrom*, Scientific Officer, SPRI, Stockholm, Sweden
*Miss N. Steel*, Senior Nursing Officer — Personnel, North Lothian
  District, Edinburgh
*Miss M.S. Stewart*, Area Nursing Officer — Personnel, Fife Health
  Board, Dunfermline, Scotland
*Miss B.M. Stocking*, Research Fellow, Nuffield Provincial Hospitals
  Trust, London
*Mrs J.E.M. Streeter*, Area Nursing Officer, Kensington and Chelsea and
  Westminster Area Health Authority, London
*Miss M.E. Thorogood*, District Nursing Officer, Grampian Health
  Board — West District, Elgin, Moray, Scotland
*Mr A. Thwaites*, Nursing Officer — Rehabilitation, Princess
  Margaret Rose Orthopaedic Hospital, Edinburgh
*Miss B. Tierney*, Chairman, Working Party on General Nursing,

Department of Health, Dublin, Ireland

*Miss J. Tinch*, Education Officer (Nursing), Scottish Health Service Centre, Edinburgh

*Mrs A. Vislie*, Research sociologist, Norwegian Hospital Institute, Trondheim

*Mrs M. Walbank*, Nursing Officer — In-service Training, Sefton Area Health Authority — Northern District, Southport, Merseyside, England

*Miss M. Walker*, Senior Nursing Officer — Post Basic Education, Northamptonshire Area School of Nursing, Wellingborough, England

*Mr B. Watkin*, Health Services Management Training, School of Business Studies, University of Manchester, England

*Miss E.M. Welsh*, Director of Nursing and Midwifery Education, Northern Ireland Council for Nurses and Midwives, Belfast

*Miss E.W. West*, Senior Nursing Officer, St Philip's Hospital, London

*Miss M. Yeo*, Nursing Officer, Welsh Office, Cardiff, Wales

Comparative International Table: Length of Training

| | Austria | Belgium | Canada | Denmark | Finland | France | Germany | Netherlands |
|---|---|---|---|---|---|---|---|---|
| 2¾ – 3½ years | RN | RN (Graduate) RN (Certificated) | RN (University) | RN | RN | RN | RN | Professional Nurse |
| 1½ – 2 years | — | Assistant · Nurse 2 years | RN (School) | — | — | — | — | Practical Nurse |
| 1 year | — | — | Certified Nursing Assistant (10 months) | Nursing Assistant | Auxiliary Nurse | Aide-Soignante | Assistant Nurse | |
| Unqualified | Auxiliary | Auxiliary | Nursing Assistant/Aide | — | Hospital Assistant (Domestic) | — | Other Nursing Personnel | |

Comparative International Table: Length of Training (Continued)

| | Norway | Portugal | Spain | Sweden | Switzerland | UK |
|---|---|---|---|---|---|---|
| 2½ – 4 years | RN | RN | RN | RN | RN | RN |
| 1½ – 2 years | – | Auxiliary Nurse (1½ years) | Practical Nurse (2 years) | – | Practical Nurse | Enrolled Nurse |
| 1 year | Nursing Assistant | – | – | Enrolled Nurse | Trained Auxiliary | – |
| Unqualified | Unqualified Auxiliary | – | Aide (waiting to start practical nurse training) | Nursing Auxiliary 6 months. Also special training from age 16 to Aide to Enrolled Nurse to RN | Untrained Auxiliary | Nursing Auxiliary |

# INDEX